FOR A BETTER MONDAY

HEALING, CLARITY, AND PURPOSE

MY JOURNEY OF FASTING AND SELF-DISCOVERY

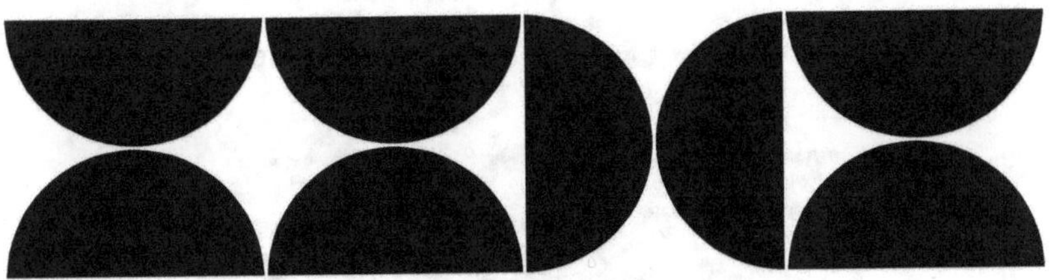

ALİ DENİZ ÖZKAN

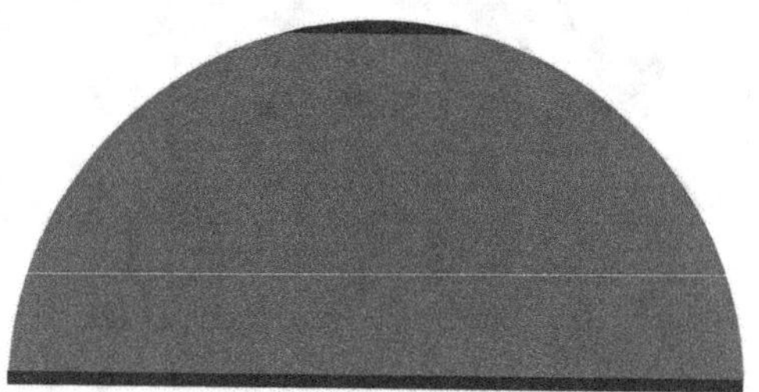

Stefan Prodanovic - Book Cover Design

Chrissy Cutting - Line Editing

Oseyi Okoeguale - Formatting & Book Interior Design

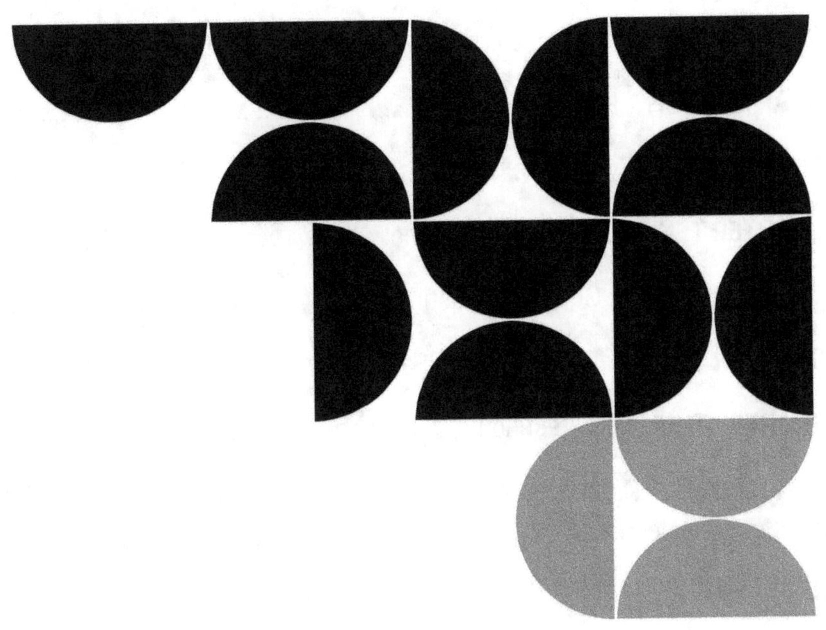

CONTENTS

CONTENTS

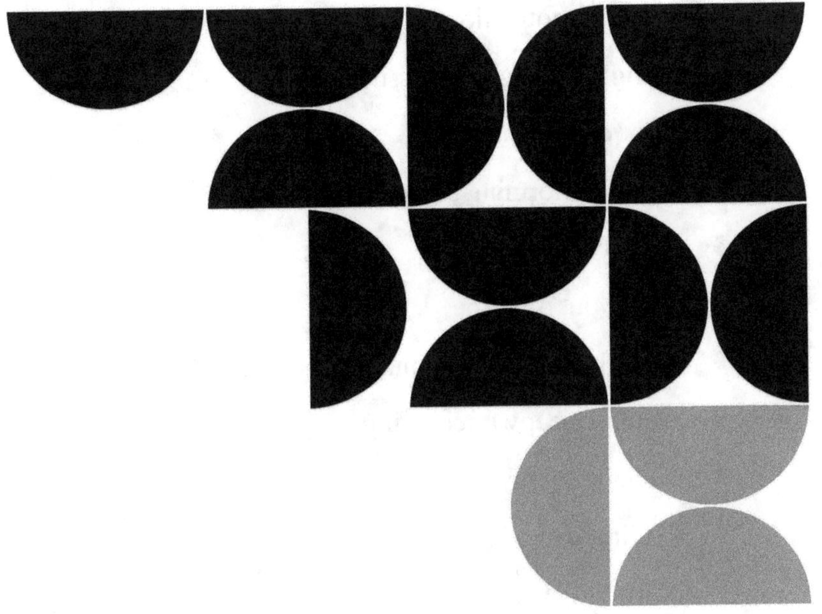

FOREWORD

For *A Better Monday* is a book about my fasting experience. I am just a regular person without any degree or certification in a health-related field, and I haven't written a book before this one. However, since incorporating fasting into my life in 2016, I have experienced significant physical, mental, and spiritual changes. With this book, I want to share my personal experience with others so we can stop wasting time on health issues and focus on our life's mission.

WHO WILL BENEFIT FROM THIS BOOK?

If you are suffering from:

- Chronic health issues
- Depression

- Lack of motivation
- Weight management issues
- Poor quality sleep
- Underperforming at work
- Lack of focus
- Being out of shape
- Negative thoughts spinning in your head
- Getting sleepy after eating
- Lack of energy
- Feeling overwhelmed
- Short attention span
- Lack of willpower

If you are addicted to sugar, social media, alcohol, porn, tobacco, carbohydrates, or compulsive money spending, *For A Better Monday* is a book for you!

This book is a comprehensive resource that can help you address multiple pain points, from chronic health issues to addiction. If any of these issues resonate, then this book is worth your time.

If you think things are going well in your life but want to improve and optimize certain areas, this book is also for you.

Fasting can be a powerful tool for solving our problems and improving in all areas of life. By harnessing the potential for self-actualization found in this book, you can transform into a better version of yourself.

HOW TO READ THIS BOOK?

While reading this book cover to cover is beneficial, it's designed to empower you to start your fasting journey as quickly as possible. Each chapter stands alone, allowing you to read specific information when needed. While some of the content may be repeated from time to time, this is to reinforce the key concepts that should be remembered during our fasting journey. The book's structure gives you the power to navigate your fasting journey at your own pace and according to your needs.

The only must-read chapters are the ones that initiate our fasting journey (Chapters 1 to 12). They are the stepping stones that lay the foundation of fasting, guiding us on the right path and providing us with the tools to improve various aspects of our lives. So, read those for sure.

Once you have the basics down, you can jump between chapters as a reader and get the needed information at the right time on your fasting journey.

If reading 12 short chapters is still too much, you can jump-start your journey by only reading Chapter 5: How to Get Started With Fasting, Chapter 11: Going Into Fasting, and Chapter 12: Coming Out of Fasting.

Chapters that provide background about myself, the author of this book, are entirely optional (From Chapter 49 to the end of the book). They serve to humanize the fasting experience further and help you relate to the challenges and triumphs of another individual. Feel free to engage with these chapters as much or as little as you like.

It can also be an option to read the chapter about the author first. That would make more sense when I refer to different places where

I have lived, such as San Diego, Switzerland, Türkiye, and Latin America. As I write this in 2024, I have spent my life on four continents and have lived as a nomad for the past eight years.

Consider this book as your fasting guide and companion. Once you've grasped the basics, you can select a chapter and turn it into your next fasting challenge or project. For instance, you can read the chapter on saving money with fasting, apply that approach to your journey, and see where it takes you.

Remember, there is no failing with fasting; there is only time passing by between two fasts. It should be an exciting and fun journey. I want you to approach this book with the same mindset. There's no pressure to finish it; instead, let the excitement of learning and the fun of constructing the new you guide your reading experience.

One could read only one chapter of this book and start their fasting journey. If the person is in tune with how their body guides them, the journey will follow without outside information. I don't claim that all the information and concepts in this book are 100% my own. However, I guarantee that everything I share has been filtered through my own personal experience. If there is something I haven't personally experienced, I will share examples of how it could work in theory.

The primary motivation behind writing and publishing this book is to inspire you through my own experiences to begin your own fasting journey. In this first edition, I have not included specific references, but I have been influenced by Thierry Casasnovas, Dr. Eric Berg, Andrew Huberman, and Dr. David Sinclair in starting my fasting journey and exploring human physiology. As I mentioned before, while not all the ideas, practices, and information in this book are original, my experiences and the results are.

As you begin *For A Better Monday*, remember that the power to transform your life lies within you. Fasting has been a transformative tool for me, and I wrote this book to share that story with you, hoping to inspire and guide you toward a healthier and more fulfilling life.

Whether you're struggling with health challenges, seeking to break free from addictions, or simply wanting to optimize your daily life, the strategies in this book can serve as your roadmap to a better version of yourself. Start where you feel the need is greatest, and let the chapters guide you.

Now is the time to take the first step. Your journey to a better Monday—and a better life—begins now. Unlock the incredible potential that fasting can bring to every aspect of your life. Let's get started.

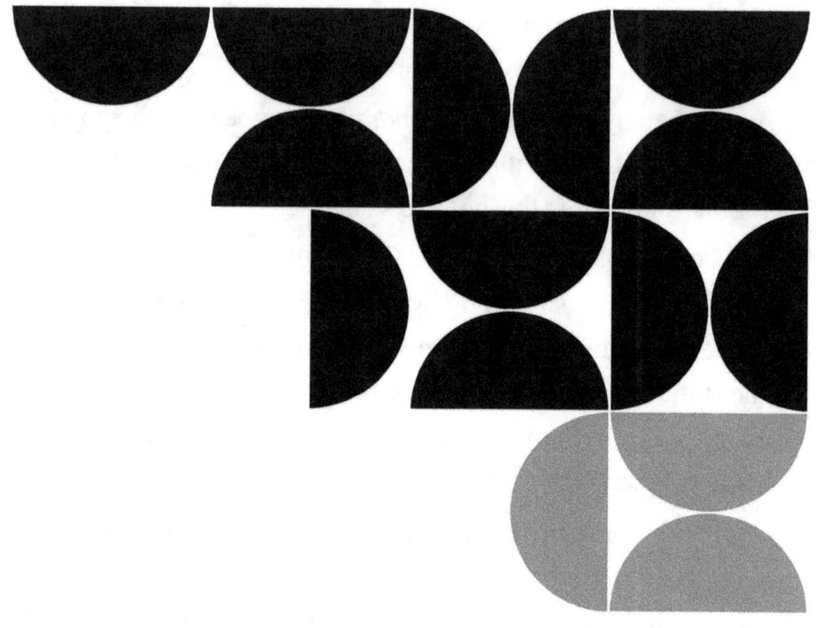

DISCLAIMER

LEGAL DISCLAIMER

The information in this communication has not been evaluated by Health Canada nor the FDA and is not intended to treat, diagnose, cure, or prevent any disease. This information is not a substitute for a qualified healthcare professional's advice or medical care. You should seek the advice of your healthcare professional before undertaking any dietary or lifestyle changes. The material provided in this communication is for educational purposes only. Every effort is made to ensure this information is accurate and as up-to-date as possible.

WARNING MESSAGE

This book is a personal account of my journey toward a healthier lifestyle, shared with a wider audience. It is important to note that I am not a health professional, nor do I possess any academic credentials in health. Therefore, I do not provide any health advice or recommendations. If you wish to try the practices that have benefited me, it is essential to adapt them to your own situation and seek professional advice. What works for me may not work for everyone, which is why developing a personalized approach based on your current health status is crucial.

I want to make it clear that I do not engage in debates about which health practices are superior. I am not concerned about the opinions of specific individuals, be they doctors or gurus. My approach is based on personal research, experimentation, and experience. If a practice has worked for me, it means it has worked for me, not necessarily for everyone. I do not claim to possess the absolute truth on any health-related topic. I have been practicing fasting since 2016 and continue to learn every day.

WHO SHOULD NOT FAST

Anybody can fast, but breastfeeding women should avoid fasting since fasting could stop breast milk production. I don't see any need for children to fast either. If you are heavily on medication, talk to your doctor first. Cutting medication abruptly could have negative consequences. If you feel too weak to start fasting, there is a chapter in this book called "Fasting May Be Too Challenging for You at First." The approach discussed in the chapter may help. I am not sure if it's okay for pregnant women to fast. If you are pregnant and want to fast, do your research. If you have any fear or doubt, or the idea of fasting makes you nervous, you should wait. A whole chapter in this book is dedicated to this topic called "The Only Danger With Fasting." Reading that chapter could be an excellent start to dissipate the fear of fasting.

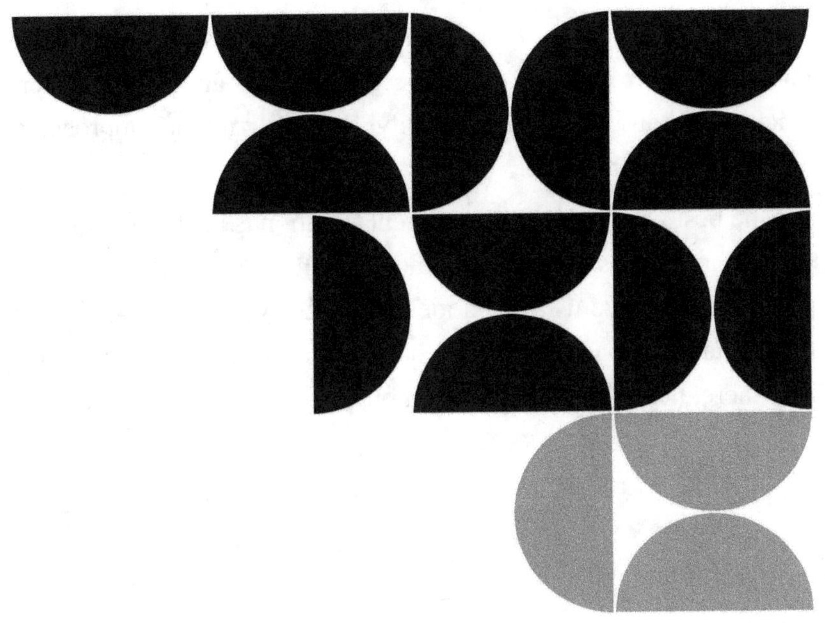

THERE IS NO SET FORMULA OR PROTOCOL FOR FASTING

Often, when I share my fasting experience in a social setting, I get the question, "How many hours should I fast?" I don't have a precise answer to that question. I am not a big believer that we are all different, but we are not all at the same place in our journey with health. There are so many factors at play, such as genetics, life hygiene, activity, and habits, that it is impossible to have a set formula for fasting.

Therefore, I suggest first assessing our current situation. We can start building from there once we know more about our current toxicity level and adaptation capacity. Personalizing our approach is the crucial element here.

The best way to assess our current situation is to start fasting and see the emerging symptoms and how much we can fast. These two indicators will give us a good idea of the body's toxicity levels and our adaptation capacity. Once we have that information, we can build from there, healing the body and improving our ability to adapt.

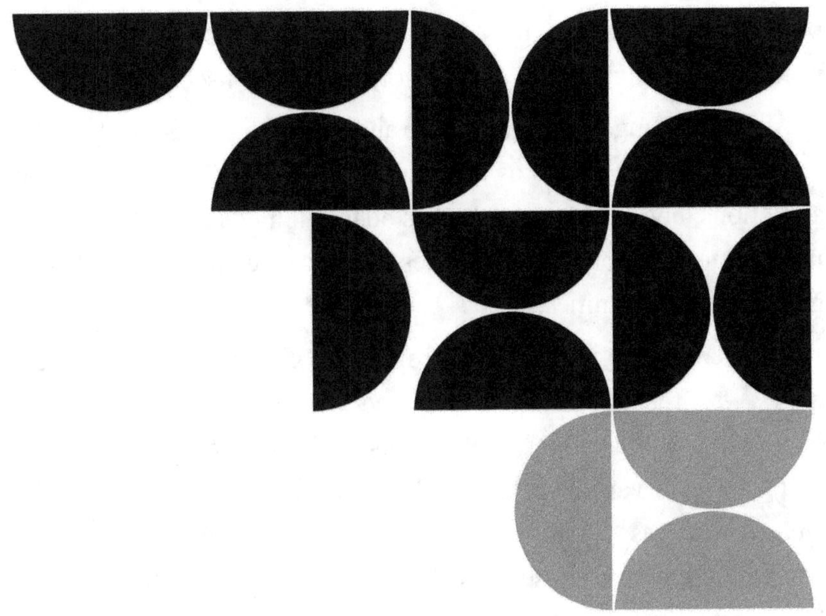

LETTING THE PROCESS HAPPEN

We find ourselves in an era where modern medicine reigns supreme in the Western world, offering quick fixes to all of our health issues. However, it's important to remember that nature operates on its own timeline, and our bodies are a part of this natural order. While modern medicine is adept at making symptoms vanish, it must often address the underlying root causes.

Fasting is a process, and things will not happen overnight. Once we start fasting regularly, the human body will begin a series of processes to return to its initial settings and repair itself. These processes take time and will occasionally create discomfort.

While fasting may require time and effort, the long-term benefits are significant. It allows us to regulate blood sugar, break free from addictions, and enhance our body's adaptation capacity. Though not immediate, these processes are a testament to the power of our body's natural healing abilities.

For example, in the first 16 months of fasting, I experienced heavy gas release from the top and bottom parts of my body. Gradually, the gas release phenomenon disappeared. My body was going through various processes to repair and cleanse itself, which created the gas situation. After regularly fasting, the body has completed these processes, and I no longer experience heavy gases. I am confident my body is functioning better now, thanks to completing these processes.

The results may take time to occur, but they will eventually. For all these reasons, it is essential to have faith in nature and see fasting as an investment.

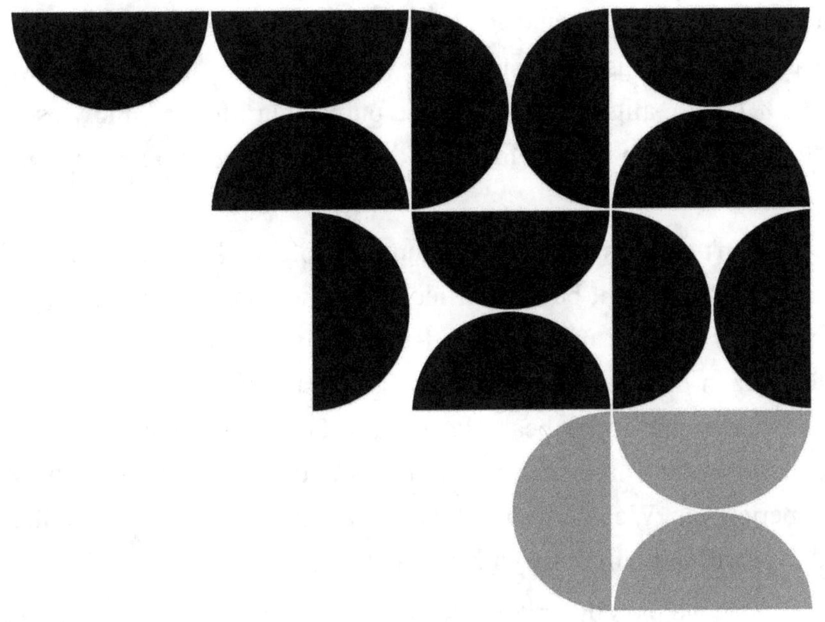

TURNING FASTING INTO A SWISS ARMY KNIFE–LIKE TOOL

We must do the groundwork before enjoying the benefits of fasting and using it as a potent tool in various areas of our lives.

The most challenging stage of fasting is the very beginning. And unfortunately, many quit at this stage. To pursue our fasting journey, we must pass this very challenging initial stage and turn fasting into a Swiss Army knife-like tool to solve almost all our life problems. Yes, fasting is that powerful. It can cure any disease, allowing us to make better decisions and answer profound spiritual questions of life. Fasting is a holistic practice that will eventually help us achieve 100% health, align us with our true purpose in life, and allow us to stop suffering so we can focus on doing the job we are meant to do on this planet.

I can't emphasize how important it is to pass the initial stages of fasting. Why can it be that difficult when we start fasting? A lot of processes will be triggered, and if we have accumulated a lot of toxicity in our body and mind throughout the years, the symptoms can be extreme and unbearable at times. Therefore, we need to have a mindset that embraces the hardship and symptoms we will be experiencing. We must believe that we are on the right track and that things will only improve with fasting time.

Once we pass the initial stages of fasting, the body has cleansed itself, our blood sugar is more regulated, and our metabolism is strengthened. We can now start fasting to increase productivity, weight management, physical and mental performance, and prevent and cure disease.

We must go through several fasting cycles to be ready to use fasting as a tool.

To conclude this chapter, we all know the saying, "What does not break you makes you stronger." A general rule of thumb with fasting is to challenge ourselves enough without breaking. Therefore, getting a good idea of our limits is crucial first. Always start small and see how the body reacts.

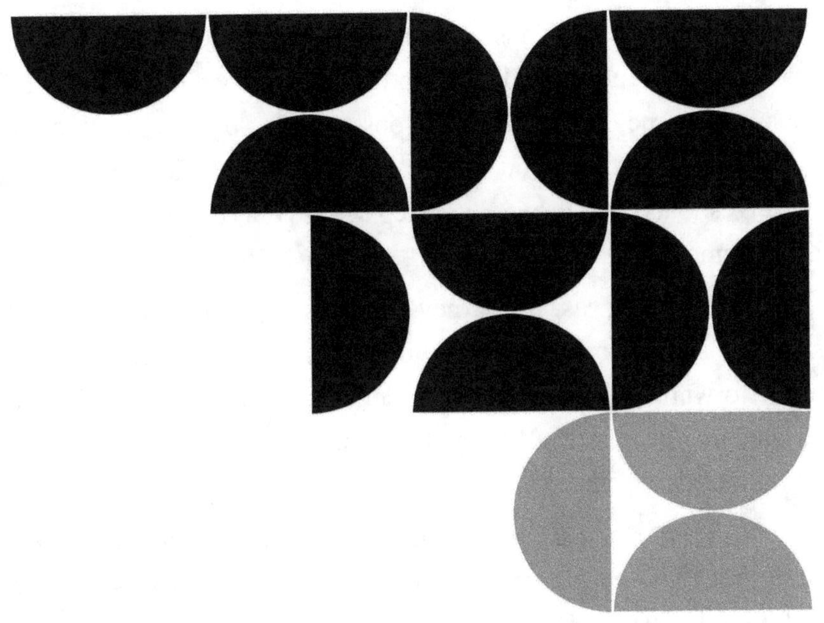

BUILDING OUR CUSTOM-MADE AND ADAPTATIVE FASTING STRATEGY

Fasting is very simple but also complex. Its complexity comes from the fact that a set recipe for success has yet to be developed. Therefore, I am skeptical when I hear people sharing protocols and formulas for perfection. We need to go further. We must build our own custom-made adaptative fasting strategy incorporating journaling, protocols, techniques, tools, patterns, and, most importantly, our fasting experience. My approach offers more of a framework to allow each individual to build their fasting journey.

The true beauty of fasting lies in its ability to foster personal growth. No two people will react to fasting exactly alike, making it a personal journey. It starts with observation, progresses through overcoming hurdles, and leads to a deeper understanding of ourselves. Each step forward is a step toward our unique path of self-improvement.

I see fasting as a journey, but that journey is far from straightforward. Sometimes, we will pause, taking steps backward to move forward later. We need to understand what to do and when to let the body express itself through fasting and learn to listen to what our bodies have to say.

One key element of building our custom-made adaptative strategy is that we are here for the long run, and there is no such thing as failing in fasting. Each fast is a new lesson. We fast and observe what is happening; when the challenge is too great, we stop, rest, and come back to fasting at a future time.

Somewhere in our minds, we need to anchor an imaginary destination. That destination is 100% health, becoming the best version of ourselves, and achieving transcendence with our life's mission. This paradise-like destination is our promised land. We need to put it somewhere in our minds, and no matter what happens and how difficult things get, always remember that this is our destination. Every attempt that we make from this moment forward is to get closer to that destination.

As we gain experience with fasting and get to know ourselves better, we can develop the strategy further. Just like in a soccer game, you cannot base your entire strategy on a protocol or technique. You have to see how the opponent or the enemy reacts to your plan to evaluate it and adapt it to the situation to make progress.

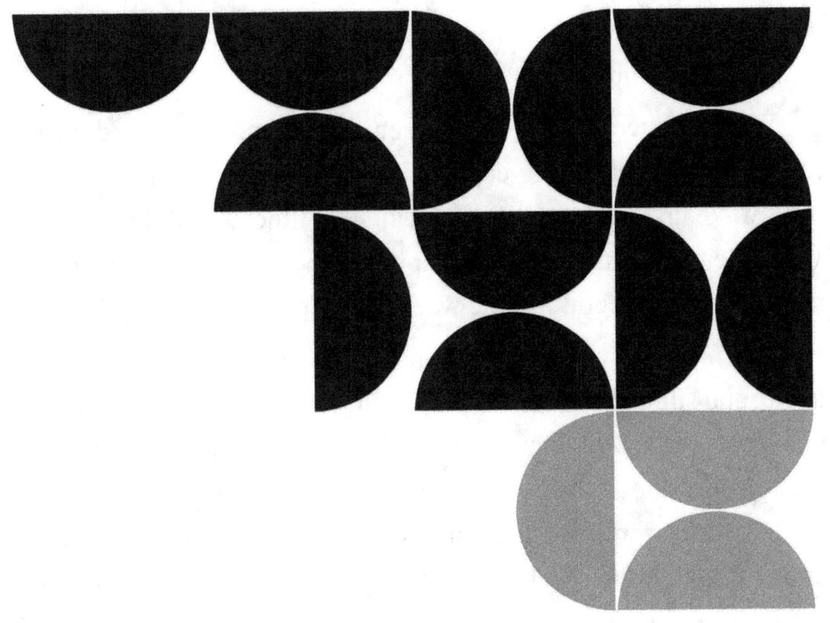

HOW TO GET STARTED WITH FASTING (1ST & 2ND TECHNIQUES)

As a fervent advocate of fasting, I've made it a lifestyle choice. This personal journey has led me to numerous conversations about fasting, often starting with the question, "How can I begin fasting?"

The answer is as easy as starting right here, right now. One can get started without anything at all. With experience, though, considering that some experience intense symptoms during detoxification, I came up with two different approaches to ease the process into fasting.

With both techniques, before getting started, it is a good idea to assess our current fasting capital. If we sleep eight hours a day and don't wake up to eat something during that time, we all already have at least eight hours of fasting capital. I recommend observing our relationship with food for one week.

When we first start eating on a given day, we write the hour down, and similarly, when we stop eating for that same day, we write it down as well. Doing this for a week will give us a good idea of our eating and fasting windows. Once we have that information in hand, we have a starting point. Many people intermittently fast without knowing they have already been fasting without making any conscious effort.

FIRST TECHNIQUE

Once we have assessed how many hours we are already fasting, the idea is to progressively increase the fasting window and decrease the food intake window. For example, if we already naturally fast 10 hours a day, we could use a weekly pattern where we fast 10 hours a day for four days, intend to fast for 12 hours for two, and have a free day where we eat and drink whenever we feel like. Then, we could replace one of the days 10 hours of fasting the following week with 12.

We will have three days of fasting for 12 hours, three for 10, and one free day. The following week, we can replace one more 10-hour fasting day with 12. Once we reach six days of fasting with 12 hours, we could fast for 14 hours the following week for one day, have five days with 12 hours of fasting, and have one off day from fasting.

With this approach, we can progressively increase our fasting window. Keep in mind that progress with fasting is sometimes linear. If you get a kick out of improving your record, keep going, but if you get bored or don't feel like fasting, feel free to take weeks off. Periods without fasting are as important as fasting. It is when we are resting that we are making progress.

SECOND TECHNIQUE

The second technique consists of choosing a day with few responsibilities and commitments. The idea is to continue fasting right after waking up and keep fasting as much as possible. When we start feeling symptoms, we can lie down, bite the bullet, and continue our fast. Once the symptoms become unbearable, we can break our fast and write down how many hours we were able to fast from our last meal.

After breaking the fast, we return to our comfort zone and continue with our life. After a few days, a week, or a couple of weeks, we can do this practice again and see how much longer we can fast and how intense the symptoms are this time. Again, once the symptoms start becoming too fierce, we can break our fast, return to our comfort zone for a time, and come back to all-day fasting later. The idea is to fast several days a month and monitor our progress.

The first technique can be smoother, and we can progress while feeling less discomfort. The second technique is more challenging, but right from the first fast, we can get a good idea of our limits so we can jump into longer fasts.

Providing a set formula is complicated because each individual has different toxicity levels and metabolism strengths. This is the reason why it is essential to evaluate our existing levels before jumping into a protocol. The idea is to find the sweet spot where fasting is becoming challenging for us and build our progress from there.

Think of it as the first training session of a soccer camp. First, they do a series of assessment tests to determine the current fitness level of all players and then assign each player an individual training program.

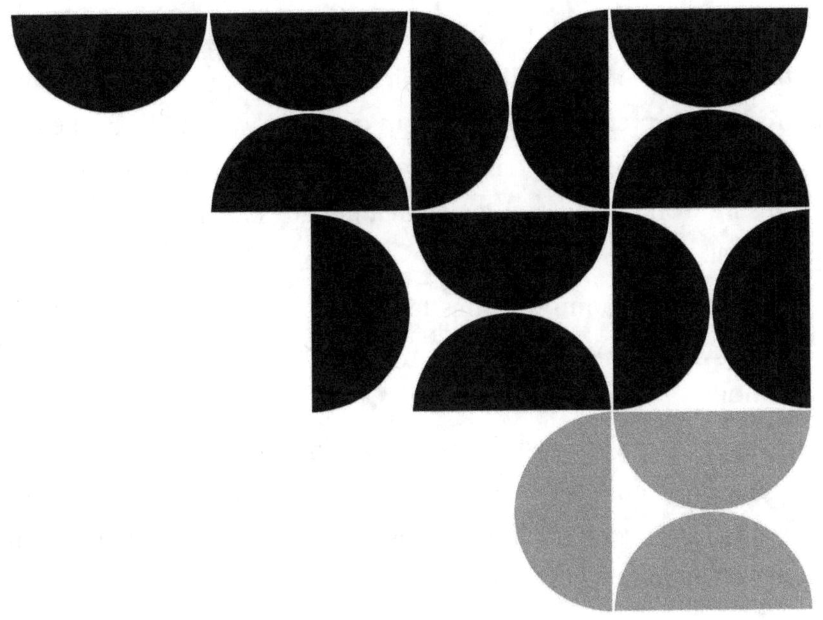

THIRD TECHNIQUE (BONUS)

If the two techniques for getting started with fasting discussed in the previous chapter sound daunting, the following technique can be used as an intermediary stage, reassuring us that we can gradually prepare our bodies for fasting.

This technique consists of changing our eating schedule and only consuming food when hungry. We should avoid snacking and never eat unless we are hungry. Our meals should be as healthy as possible, made of whole foods, and exclude processed foods as much as possible.

This technique will train our ability to listen to our body, which is the most important skill to acquire for our fasting journey. If we correctly interpret the messages from our body, we will be pushed to fast naturally. Generally, if the body is busy doing its repair and cleansing work, then it will not signal hunger so that it can finish its tasks first.

The rule of thumb with this technique is never to eat if you are not hungry and to distinguish between the signals of hunger and addiction.

If you start your fasting journey with this technique, the skill you'll develop during this early stage will help you throughout. Not eating when we don't feel hungry is a straightforward rule that can have tremendous positive effects.

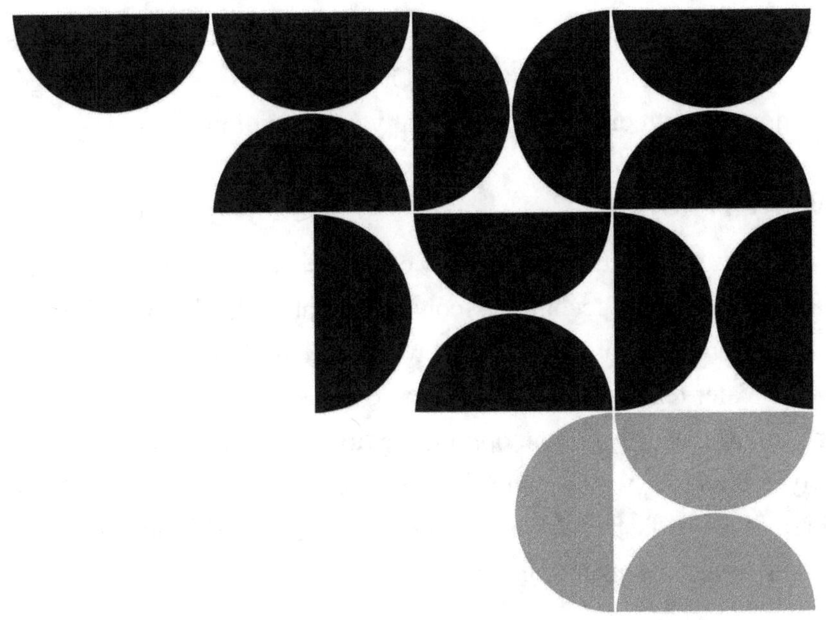

DIFFERENT TYPES OF FASTS

There are different ways to fast. I see them as tools in my journey to well-being. One is not better than another. They are distinct and can be used according to the situation.

DRY FASTING

I have the most experience with this type of fast, which consists of not consuming any food or liquid. It may sound like the most challenging way of fasting, but it is easier for me to dry fast than water fast. It is a fast that will go deeper in cleansing. Since the body is deprived of water, it will find ways to find some, triggering a series of actions inside our bodies. One could experience stronger symptoms with dry fasting, especially in the beginning.

WATER FASTING

As its name indicates, we only consume water when we are water fasting. Different techniques could be applied to this fast. It's not because we are water fasting that we should drink abundant water all day. Water tends to dilute blood and can make us dizzy. The fasting period is also an excellent opportunity to give our kidneys some rest. My approach to water-fasting has been to dry fast for as long as I can, breaking my fast with some water near nighttime, and then keep going without consuming too much water.

FASTING WITH ELECTROLYTES

I discovered fasting with electrolyte supplements when my business mentor suggested it as a niche product to sell online. At first, I was skeptical because I firmly believed that we didn't need external support to fast. However, when I incorporated electrolyte supplements into my water fasts, it worked amazingly well. When we water fast, we lose some fasting functionalities compared to dry fasting. However, water-fasting with electrolyte supplements is an excellent solution for getting going with our day and being active and productive. I eventually created my own electrolyte company, YouthLyte. I incorporated fasting with electrolytes into my fasting routine when I am water fasting, preparing for a long dry fast, or coming out of it. If you plan on using electrolyte supplements during your fast, make sure that the powder you use does not have any sweetener or flavoring. YouthLyte has a product called "Fasting

Electrolytes," which is free of any sweeteners or flavoring. In addition to the foremost electrolytes, it has a compound of 72 trace minerals.

LOW-CALORIE LIQUID FASTING

This fast consists of not consuming any solid food and only consuming tea, coffee, matcha, sugarless electrolyte water, and occasionally hot water cacao. I've come up with this fasting protocol to accompany me during the writing process of this book. It has worked perfectly well so far. I've been skipping my OMAD once to twice a week. It means only eating five to six meals a week. I've been fasting this way on Wednesdays and Saturdays. On Thursdays and Sundays, I usually wake up with lots of energy.

What I love about this fast is that I can still go to coffee shops and coworking spaces to get some work done. Another aspect I love about this fast is that I've been working on my projects seven days a week without feeling any fatigue. Fasting on Saturdays still makes the weekend feel different, and on Monday, I've been starting the week refreshed. After only fasting on Saturdays, I added Wednesday to be even more productive. Everything has its limits. I don't see myself fasting like this forever.

The only downside I could see to this process is consuming lots of coffee and tea on an empty stomach. I did not experience any issues, but it could irritate people with weaker stomachs.

After fasting twice a week for over 40 days, I returned to fasting this way only on Wednesdays. My body communicated to me that it needed more eating days to recuperate. As I write this, I have completed two months of fasting this way. It has been outstanding in terms of productivity and the pleasure of working.

JUICE FASTING

A fasting approach could be only to consume juices for a set period. One would lose many of the functionality and benefits of fasting by juice-fasting, but since we are not consuming solid food during a juice fast, the digestive system is still getting a break. It can rest and regenerate.

We should be careful not to juice excessive amounts of fruits that can contain high sugar. Juicing should be made of a high percentage of vegetables and elements that support circulation and cleansing, such as ginger, turmeric, and garlic.

Juice fasting could be a favorable stepping stone for those intimidated by dry or water fasting.

MONO MEALS

This approach is technically not a fast anymore because we will be eating some solid food, but the fact that we only consume one ingredient per meal gives a break to many digestive functions. As with juice fasting, mono meals could ease into fasting progressively for those who don't want to do the big jump into fasting immediately.

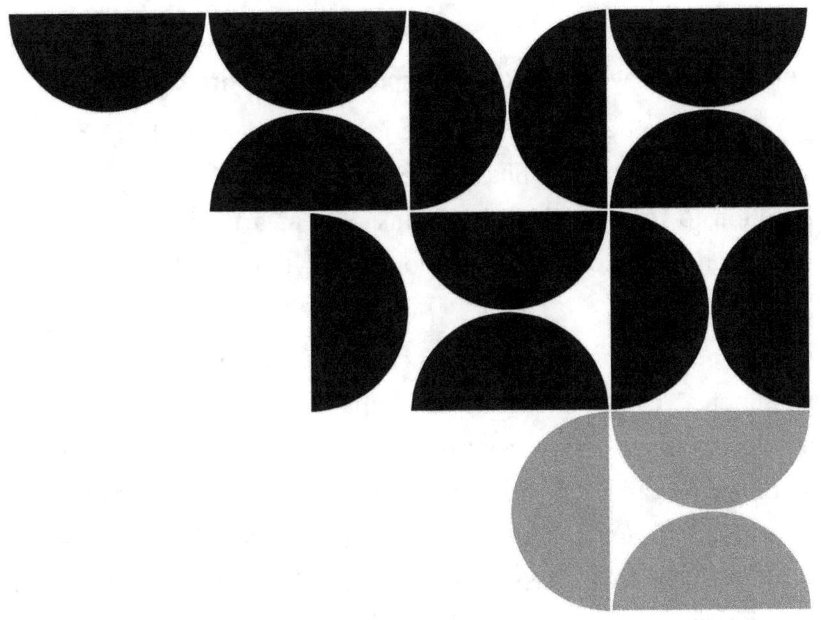

HEALING CRISES

Fasting is a fantastic journey and the best investment toward a healthier and happier life. That said, fasting isn't always easy. We will face many challenges during our fasting journey.

We must keep an open mind during fasting and see the challenges as investment opportunities. We are suffering right here, right now, to feel healthier, stronger, and happier in the future.

It is tough to predict exactly how one will feel during fasting. When we fast, we allow our body to do its thing. There will be euphoric moments when we feel lots of energy, and there will be moments when we experience symptoms or feel tired.

Typically, the discomfort experienced during a fast is a healing crisis. It's a temporary phase where our body takes a break from digestion to focus on healing. Think of it as a freeway closure for maintenance. Once the work is done, everything will run smoother than before.

The good news about healing crises is that they usually last 5 to 15 minutes. Learning to bite the bullet when they occur is good practice. If they don't go away and we feel like we can't take it anymore, we can break our fast. But biting the bullet allows the body to heal itself. Once the crisis goes away, we feel good about ourselves, as if we've passed one more hurdle toward our destination of becoming a better version of ourselves.

Another advantage of biting the bullet during a healing crisis is that it allows the body to finish the process of what it is doing. If we are experiencing a healing crisis, the body is fixing something at that moment. Interrupting the process in the middle will postpone the task until a future time. Therefore, we can better wait for the body to do its thing. Once the healing crisis is over, we can decide if we continue the fast or break it. Of course, if the symptoms are unbearable or if you feel in danger, you should never hesitate to break your fast at any time.

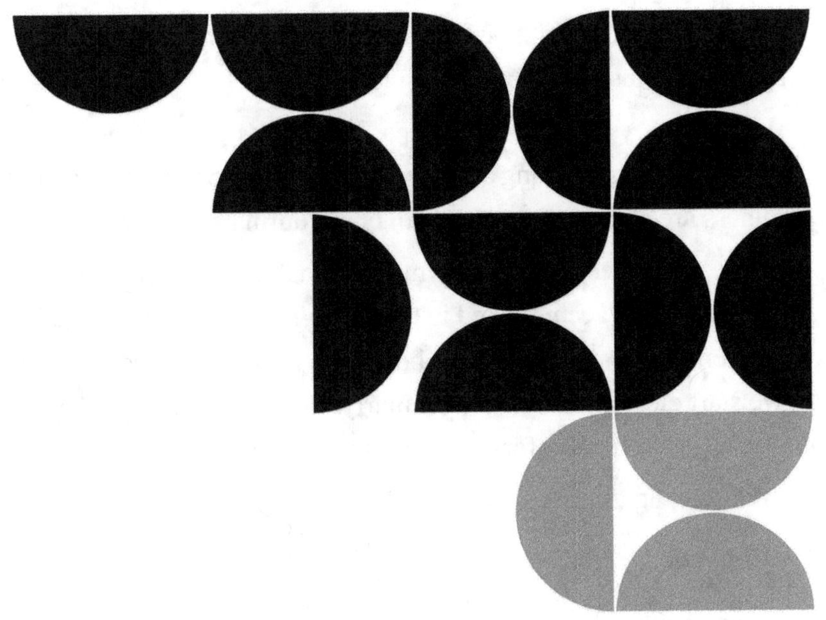

CHAPTER
NINE

SYMPTOMS WHILE FASTING

It is crucial to understand that the symptoms we experience while fasting are entirely typical. While they can be uncomfortable, they indicate that our body responds to fasting healthily.

One positive aspect of experiencing symptoms while fasting is that it clearly shows that the fasting process is working. It's a testament to the body's natural detoxification abilities.

While they can vary in intensity, these symptoms are temporary and a direct result of the body's current toxicity level. In my personal experience, my first dry fast of 36 hours was the most challenging, but subsequent fasting sessions became more manageable, with similar symptoms appearing during longer fasts.

Headaches, muscular cramps, dizziness, vomiting, skin reactions, tiredness, having a fuzzy mind, feelings of depression, and sleepiness are all symptoms that can occur during fasting.

I see the uncomfortable symptoms as a result of cleansing excessive toxicity accumulated in the body. The first cleaning session will generate dirt and dust like a house we haven't cleaned in years. As we start cleaning the house regularly, the process will get easier. It's similar to the uncomfortable symptoms of fasting.

Start fasting today!

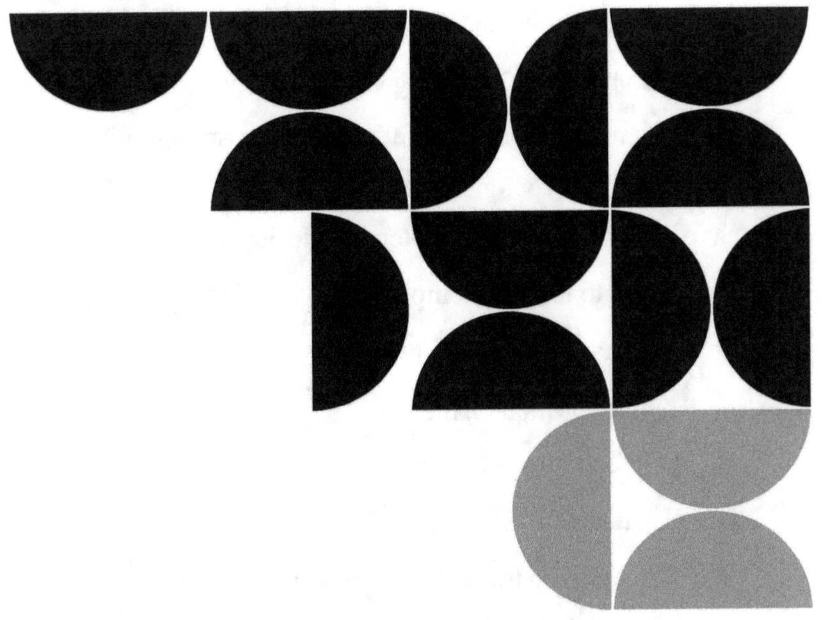

KEEP A FASTING JOURNAL

The fasting journal is a great tool to keep track of our progress. I would start the journal even before beginning the fasting experience. Write down all the things you are unhappy and struggling with in life. It could be physiological symptoms like

- I cannot get a good night's sleep,
- I suffer from hemorrhoids,
- I have allergies,
- I have eczema, or

- I have back pain.

It could also be mental challenges or conditions, such as

- I want to get rid of negative thoughts spinning in my head.

- I want to stop making terrible decisions.

- I tend to lose my temper and regret it afterward.

- I am having a hard time concentrating.

Also, list your spiritual challenges.

- Do you know why are you on this planet?

- What is your life mission?

- What do you think that is separating you from the perfect life you want to live?

Once you start fasting, log all your fasting hours and the intended fasting patterns. Write down how you feel and the symptoms you are experiencing. You must specify how far you are into the fast in your logs. An example could be,

- "I am 14 hours into my second dry fast, and I feel extremely thirsty."

  or

- "I just finished hour 16 of my dry fast, and the sensation of thirst has disappeared."

Once you have gone through several fasting cycles, returning to the journal, and comparing how you felt during a specific fast hour will allow you to track your progress, draw conclusions, and organize your next fasting steps.

The list of symptoms and discomfort you felt before starting fasting will be crucial to monitoring your progress. In my experience, many of the symptoms I was struggling with in the past have disappeared. When I think of them today, it feels like they were from a different life.

One thing that will probably happen is that the symptoms you might feel during fasting, such as headaches and cramps, may occur later in your fasting. This also proves that our adaptation capacity is increasing, and we are progressing well.

Before each fasting project, you can write down your intention. It could be something like, "This week, I intend to do an 18/6 intermittent fasting from Monday to Saturday, and on Sunday, I am going to rest from fasting." Then, you can log how you feel each day. Once the week comes to an end, you can write down how it went, whether you were able to keep up with what you had planned, and what your next fasting project is going to be.

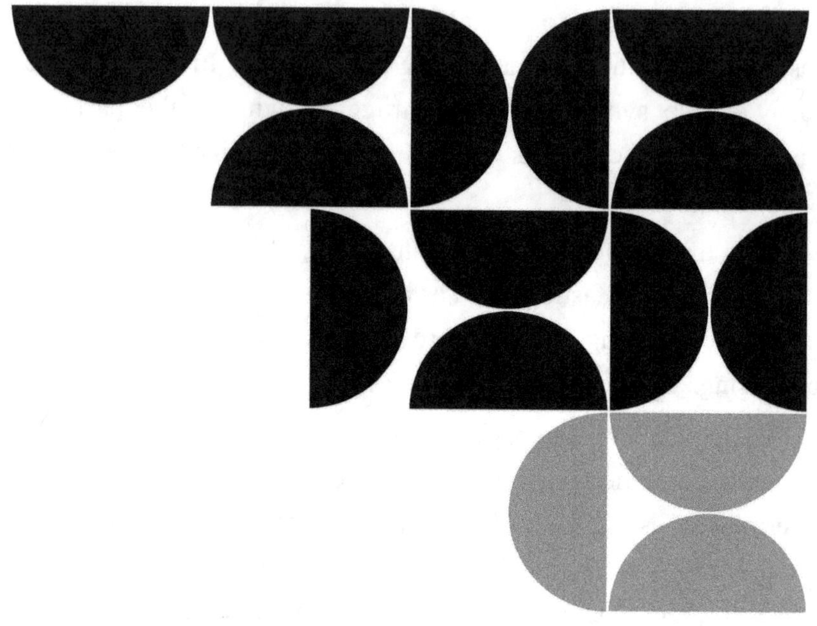

GOING INTO FASTING

In reality, we don't need to do anything in particular to go into a fast. All we have to do is stop consuming food and liquids if we are dry fasting.

Preparing can help us reap more benefits from our fasting sessions. A good strategy is to ease in. A day or two before starting our fast, we could consider only eating raw fruits and vegetables.

There are various structured approaches to fasting preparation, each offering a sense of accomplishment as we progress. For instance, starting with a day of salads, followed by a day of juice fasting, and then transitioning into a complete fast can be a motivating journey that helps the body adjust to the fasting process.

During fasting, it's important to practice self-care. Consuming electrolytes before and during fasting, especially if we are on a water or juice fast, can help us feel nurtured and cared for, ensuring our body's needs are met.

While a fast is a fast, not preparing for it can have drawbacks. Consider this scenario: your last meal before fasting is a heavy pizza. Some of your fasting time and energy will be spent digesting that heavy meal, delaying the body's cleansing and repair functions. Conversely, if we ease into fasting with lighter, easy-to-digest foods, we can make the most of our fasting time and reap better benefits.

Preparing could be a plus for starting a fast, but in my experience, it's not absolutely necessary. Especially when we have completed various fasting cycles, each individual will get a sense of the best way to start a fast. What we want to avoid is fasting because we think we haven't prepared. Any fast will be good for us. We shouldn't use not having completed the preparation period as an excuse not to fast.

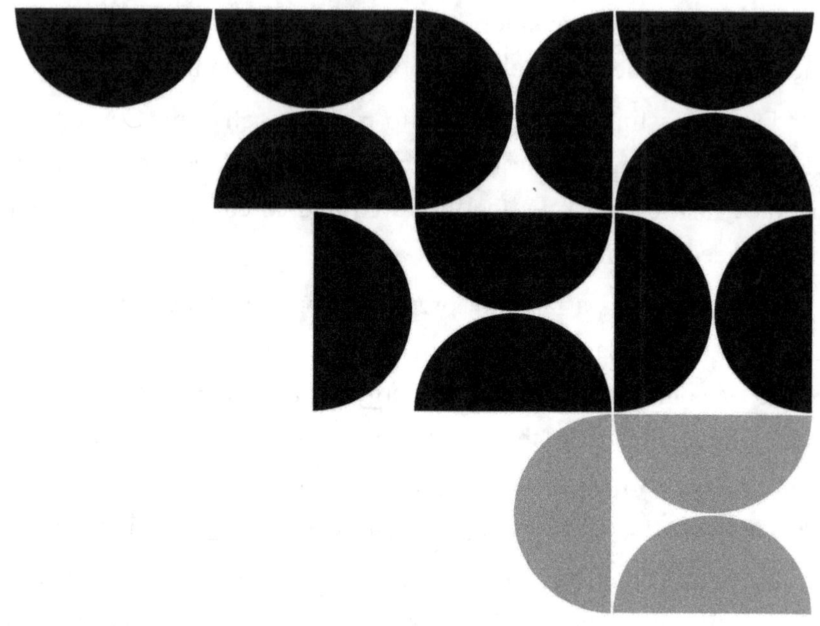

COMING OUT OF FASTING

While the techniques I've shared for entering fasting are flexible, the methods I'm about to discuss for breaking our fasts are of utmost importance and should be approached with caution.

The rule of thumb here is that the longer the fast, the more careful we need to go out of the fast.

I usually break my fast with water, coconut water, lime juice, or some electrolyte powder dissolved into water. Taking our time and not drinking large quantities of water right when breaking a fast is essential, especially if we've been dry fasting. When we dry fast, the body is in water-saving mode. If we start drinking too much of it immediately, we will experience bloating. The technique is to take only one sip of water to break the fast and wait between eight to ten minutes. This way, we signal to the body that we are breaking our fast and that food and water are coming. This approach allows time for the body to get out of water-saving mode.

I recommend consuming liquids for a while, then easy-to-digest possible raw food such as a salad. We can then slowly get back to eating normal.

If our fast was short, say 36 to 42 hours, we could adopt a progressive approach within a few hours of breaking it. However, if our fast was long, we must be more patient. After breaking my 10-day dry fast, I only consumed liquids for a few days. I then transitioned to salads for one day and steamed vegetables the next day. It took me about five days to return to eating normally.

When breaking a fast, it's crucial to avoid sugar spikes and shocks to the body. It means steering clear of foods like pizza or burgers. Instead, consider a more balanced option like lemon juice diluted in water with sugarless electrolyte powder. By being aware of these risks, we can make informed choices for our health. I don't recommend breaking a fast with high-sugar liquids such as orange juice.

Breaking a fast is a pivotal moment in the fasting cycle that demands patience and self-discipline. It's not the end of the journey where we can indulge in anything we desire. The body still requires time to readjust, and we hold the reins to guide it during this process.

A rule of thumb is that the body needs the same amount of time as it was deprived of food and water to return to its normal state after breaking the fast. If we have fasted for 72 hours, for the next 72 hours after breaking our fast, we should remember that our body is still recovering.

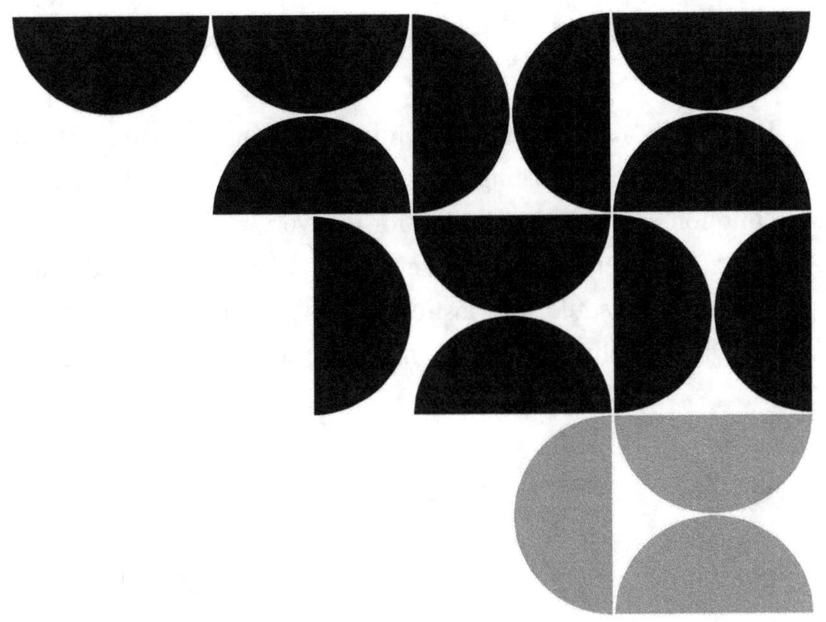

RESTING FROM FASTING

Taking a break and returning to our comfort zone is as important as fasting to reap its benefits.

A bodybuilder does not build muscular mass at the gym. At the gym, she rips the muscular tissue by applying stress. She then eats; during sleep, new muscle tissue is created, and progress is made.

Similarly, fasting follows a cycle of rest and challenge. After a fasting period, it is crucial to return to our comfort zone and enjoy the benefits. This rest period prepares us for a more challenging fast, enhancing the benefits and motivating us on our wellness journey.

I cannot stress enough that rest is crucial to getting the fasting benefits.

We usually refer to fasting as refraining from consuming food. In reality, the entire fasting cycle is when we refrain from food consumption and have equal time for recovery and returning to our comfort zone. Therefore, we will need time to recover from the fast, and so must schedule our fasting sessions accordingly. We can achieve great results by repeating the entire stress and rest cycle.

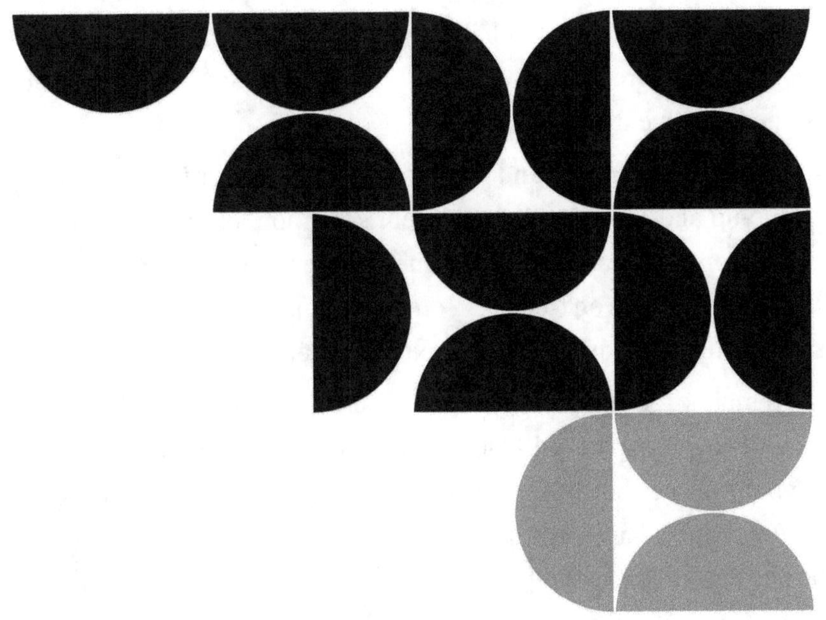

THE MORE FASTING CHALLENGES US, THE MORE WE NEED IT

I consider fasting the best thing that has happened to me. It's a miracle practice and a solution for almost all health problems.

While fasting does present its challenges, the rewards are truly worth it. It's a journey that requires effort, but the moments of struggle are not roadblocks. They are opportunities for you to prove your resilience and take control of your health. They are stepping stones to the ultimate prize—a healthier, more vibrant you.

While fasting can be challenging, particularly for those in poor health. The more severe the health issues, the longer fasts will be needed to solve them.

Intermittent fasting and shorter fasts are great for giving the body a tune-up and optimizing our current condition, but if our condition is poor and we have chronic issues, intermittent fasting and short fasting sessions won't cut it. You must train your body with those short fasting sessions to fast for extended periods later.

Think of fasting as paying off credit card debt. If we're in significant debt, we will need more than the minimum monthly payment to get out of the red. Similarly, if our health condition is severe, more than intermittent fasting or short fasting sessions may be needed. But the potential for significant health improvements with longer fasts is a beacon of hope, a light at the end of the tunnel that should inspire our determination to keep going.

If we don't feel like fasting or encounter intense symptoms as a reaction when we attempt to fast, this should not discourage us. On the contrary, it is a sign that the body needs some time off eating to repair itself. Facing challenges while fasting should motivate us. It means we are on the right path but still have a long way to go.

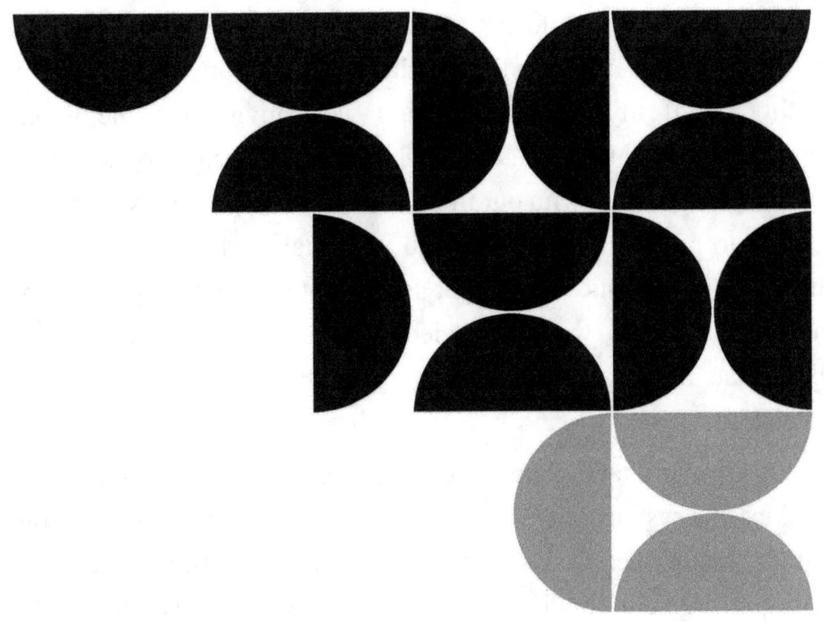

GET TO A CLEAN SLATE SITUATION

As I write this, I've been fasting for over eight years. If I compare how I interpreted my body's messages before starting my fasting journey, I see that a lot has changed.

What I interpreted as hunger and thirst before starting my fasting journey weren't real hunger and thirst. I would also interpret symptom suppression by medication as curing. Now, I know what it takes to cure an imbalance sustainably. Medication also creates side effects, which overload the message channel from the body with information that should not be there in the first place.

The point I want to get to is this: Before starting my fasting journey, I was navigating through life with a distorted perception of reality, as if my internal compass were giving me the wrong information. In such a situation, it is almost impossible to make wise decisions. It is why, with our first fasting sessions, we must bring our bodies to a clean slate situation to understand what our bodies are trying to communicate. Hunger is not your blood sugar dropping abruptly because we are loaded up with sugary items during breakfast. In reality, what we interpret as hunger, in this case, is addiction.

If we don't take control of our bodies, we will remain sort of junkies of a system that favors the food and pharmaceutical industries rather than our health. To move forward with our fasting journey, we must bring our bodies to this clean slate situation so the communication channel between our body and us is clear of noise. To achieve this, we need to regulate our blood sugar and avoid substances such as chemical-based medicine as much as possible. Of course, please consult your doctor before cutting down on any medication. More and more doctors nowadays give credit to natural healing and fasting. Having an open-minded healthcare practitioner could be a good solution.

With my journey, I quit medication altogether, and after a year, I started fasting. It worked well for me, but I did not have a severe condition, nor was I using heavy medication.

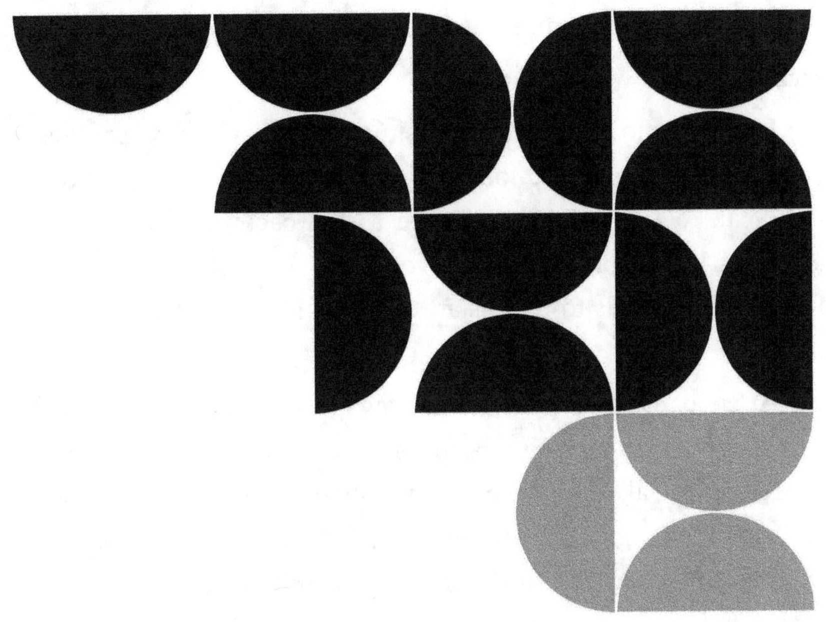

FASTING MAY BE TOO CHALLENGING FOR YOU AT FIRST

Despite the initial challenges, fasting can be a potent tool for fortifying our bodies. By overcoming the stress that fasting initially induces, we can establish a pattern where each fasting session becomes a source of strength and resilience, enhancing our overall well-being.

Listening to your body during fasting is paramount. Sometimes, your body is too fatigued and lacking in essential minerals to handle even a short fast, signaling the need to adjust your fasting routine for your safety and well-being.

I have yet to experience this situation, but with my experience and logical thinking, the following might be the solution. If we are too weak to fast, we need to take a step backward and do other activities before bringing ourselves to a level where we can start fasting. The idea is to jump-start the body like a car with a drained battery.

A good starting point is to engage in passive regenerative activities, such as massages, sauna sessions, and sunbathing. Juicing vegetables can also help when the digestive system is tired. Providing the body with high-quality nutrients that are easy to digest is a good approach. We can add fresh ginger, curcumin, garlic, and hot chili pepper to those juices for an extra boost.

Imagine an exhausted body after several massages, sunbathing, and sauna sessions drinking organic vegetable juices with natural boosting ingredients. Now, the person can try intermittent fasting and continue passive regenerative practices with juicing.

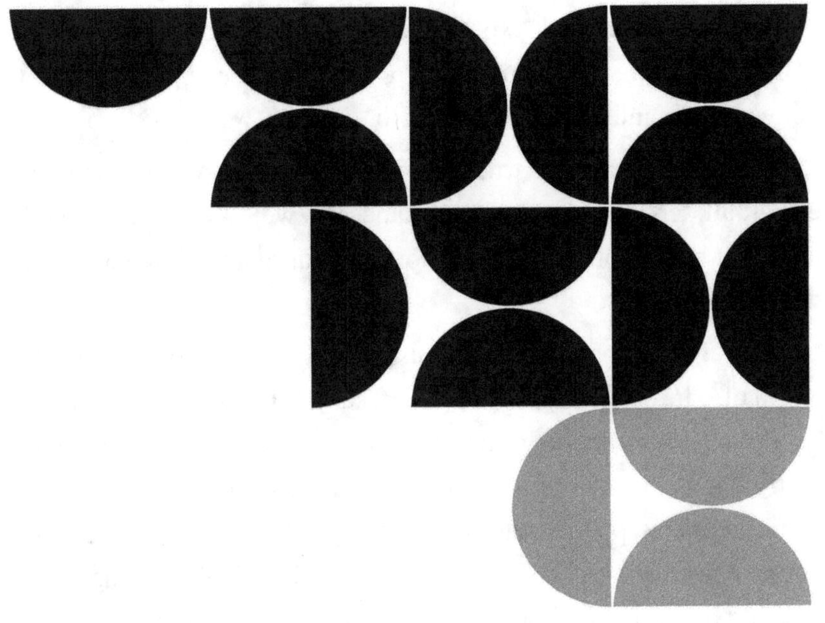

THE ONLY DANGER WITH FASTING

Before starting my fasting journey, I heard all kinds of urban legends, such as,

- "If you don't drink for three days, you will die."

- "Fasting will destroy your kidneys."

- "Fasting will dehydrate you."

- "Breakfast is the most important meal of the day."

From my personal experience, all these are lies. Those false beliefs are purposefully put out there to serve interest groups that are not genuinely interested in our health.

I admit that what is true for me may not be valid for someone else. It all depends on the circumstances as well. I could dry fast for ten days, but if you put me in a hot sauna during my dry fast, I may not last 24 hours.

It is always good to be cautious, but fasting isn't something to be afraid of. The only danger I see with fasting is to combine it with fear. If you are unsure about going into a fast, you will be stressed out and worrying the whole time. This combination could be dangerous. What separates people who die of hunger from the ones reaching optimal health is a very fine line inside the mind. Fasting is not starving because we choose to fast as opposed to starving, which is something imposed on us, but most importantly, when we fast, we have faith in fasting. We know that it is going to do us good. So, if you don't have faith or feel nervous about fasting, it's better to wait, gain knowledge, and build the missing self-confidence.

Doing research is an excellent way to gain self-confidence in fasting. The more we understand how the human body operates, the more mentally ready we will be to begin fasting. With research, we must remember that giant industries out there don't want us to fast. If we start fasting regularly and solve our health-related problems, many of those industries will go out of business. Since those industries also have some control over information, we need to keep an open mind when researching online. Searching through search results on the second, third, and fourth pages can also be beneficial.

A good approach if we experience fear could be to research until we gain enough confidence and start fasting with baby steps.

Building that faith and confidence before jumping into fasting is very important.

The only danger with fasting is fear for people within a specific norm. If you are in a particular group, such as breastfeeding or pregnant women, if you are on heavy medication, or if you have poor health, seek professional advice. Finding a doctor who is who is open-minded to fasting and alternative healing techniques is particularly helpful.

Although I see fear as the only danger of fasting, please read the chapter of this book called "Coming Out of Fasting." Breaking our fast the wrong way can also represent some danger; we could hurt ourselves if we don't break our fast correctly.

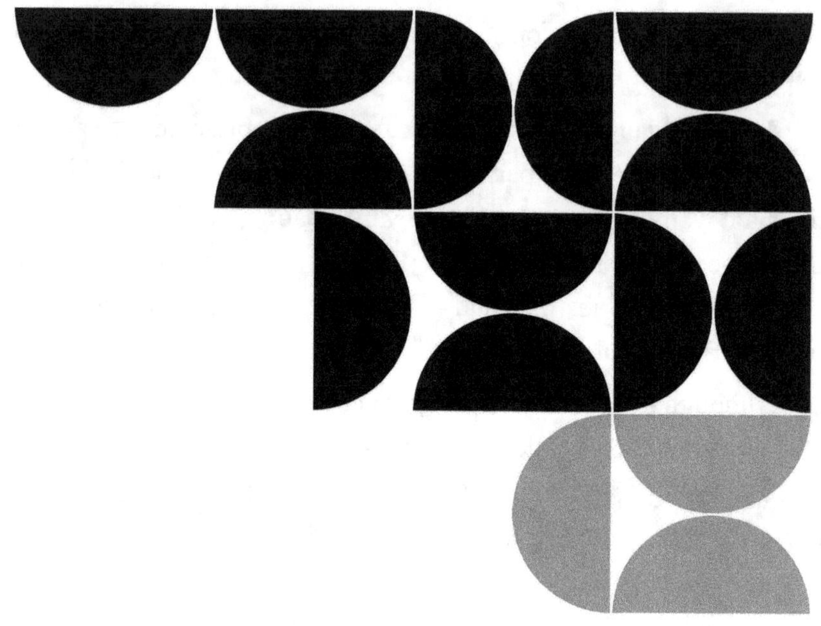

SEASONS AND ENVIRONMENTAL FACTORS WHEN FASTING

Understanding the adaptability of fasting to different seasons and environments is crucial. While these factors can pose challenges, they are not insurmountable. Recognizing their potential impact on our fasting routine is critical to making informed decisions and feeling confident in our fasting journey.

Depending on your geographical location, the weather can significantly influence your fasting experience. In regions with distinct seasons, summer and winter can introduce additional hurdles to fasting, particularly if you're new to fasting and your body needs to fully adapt to the fasting challenge.

Summers could be brutal, especially if we have decided to dry fast. Sweating can cause us to lose fluids, which will challenge us fast.

Wintertime also has its challenges. We tend to find comfort in warm food when the weather is cold. Not having that support and going through healing crises when there is less sunlight during the day can be factors that make us feel depressed.

The social aspect of fasting can also be a significant hurdle. As social interactions often revolve around food and drinks, staying focused on your fast can be a test of willpower. Fasting is already a considerable test of self-discipline, and missing out on social opportunities can make the fasting experience even more demanding.

I have lived by myself for almost a decade and a half. It was easy for me to have an environment where I could focus on fasting. If one lives with a spouse or family, and if people around them are eating three or four times a day, snacking and preparing food can be challenging for the fasting person.

It is a good idea to communicate that we are fasting to the people we live with, but even that could not be enough. In the summer of 2022, I lived with my mom for several weeks at her house in Türkiye. Every morning, she would ask me if I wanted to have breakfast. Although she knew about my lifestyle, seeing me fasting in front of her eyes made her worried, and throughout the day, she would ask me several times if I wanted to eat something. Being reminded of food from external factors can be an extra challenge.

When we refuse food, people sometimes ask us why; when we explain why, they may be surprised and ask many questions. Some will provide arguments that it is dangerous. All these unnecessary interactions can add stress to our fasting experience.

It's crucial to remember that fasting is a journey that requires resilience. Even when conditions are not ideal, we can still fast. Understanding that external factors can make fasting more or less difficult is part of the journey, and overcoming these challenges can be empowering.

In the process of writing this book, I spent the months of May and June in Medellin, Colombia. It was my fourth visit to Medellin. During the 68 days I spent there on this visit, I reached a level of productivity and well-being I had never experienced before. I was fasting one to two days a week. I could access seawater, black salt, and MCT oils in many specialized health stores. All the ketogenic-compatible berry types of foods were also available in Colombia for an affordable price.

Medellin is at the equator but in attitude. This situation results in 12 hours of sunlight and 12 hours of darkness daily. The temperature is between 25 and 29 degrees Celsius / 77 - 84 Fahrenheit year-round. Not only was the best coffee available in Colombia, but my neighborhood, Laureles, also had many coworking spaces and coffee shops that welcomed digital nomads.

All these factors, combined with going to the gym five to six times a week, made me feel like I was on top of the world, both in terms of how I physically felt and how I was getting work done.

I had to return to Asuncion in Paraguay at the end of my stay. It happened to be wintertime there. When I arrived at the airport at night, I was welcomed by a 1-degree Celsius / 32.8 Fahrenheit temperature. For ten days, the weather was cold, and less healthy food was available. It took me almost two weeks to feel great again. I even got sick when the temperature out of nowhere suddenly increased to 30 degrees Celsius / 86 degrees Fahrenheit. The air quality in Asuncion is generally also of lesser quality than in Medellin.

I am sharing this personal experience comparing two locations to emphasize the importance of the environment. I was at the top of the world health-wise and productivity-wise in one location. Switching countries and seasons affected me greatly. Even though I had developed a high adaptability capacity with fasting and constantly traveling, my output and feelings weren't the same when many factors in my environment changed.

As I write these lines, I have been in Asuncion for almost a month, and I am doing fantastic. However, I am a bit below productivity in comparison to my last stay in Medellin.

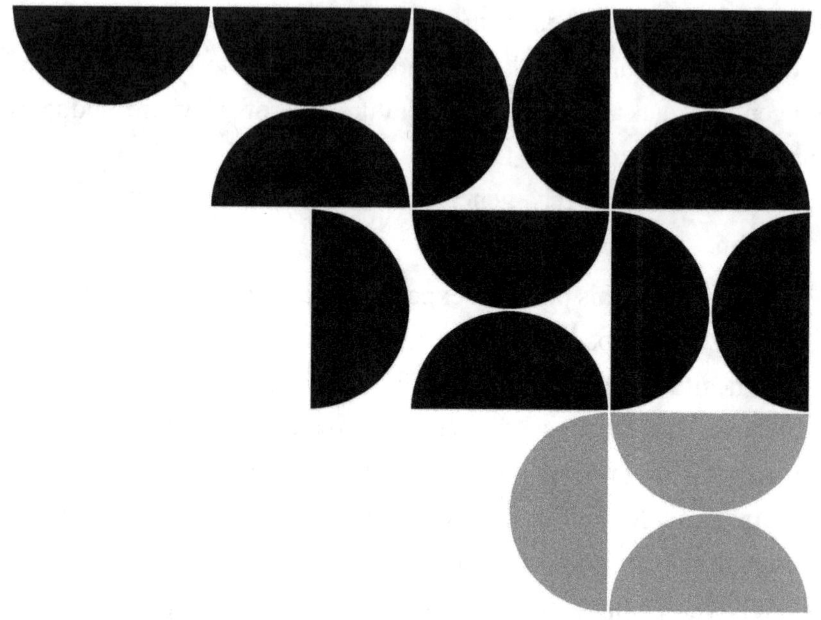

WILL FASTING MAKE US LOSE WEIGHT?

Many wonder if fasting can aid in weight loss. It's disheartening to see that the focus is often on appearance rather than health. However, when it comes to fasting, the answer is more complex than yes or no. When done right, fasting can have numerous health benefits, including weight loss.

It is evident that going into a fast puts us in a caloric deficiency state, and we lose some weight. But once we break our fast and go back to eating regularly, we will gain the weight we have lost.

If we fast regularly, we will eventually reach our ideal weight. It means someone who is overweight will lose weight, and someone who is very skinny may gain weight. The idea is that fasting will bring our bodies back to our factory settings. If we are overweight, there is most likely a physiological reason. The same goes if we are way too skinny. It may come from a food absorption problem in the colon. In both situations, fasting will help to bring us closer to our ideal weight.

What is essential to consider is that fasting is not a diet. Even though we restrict ourselves from food during a portion of our fasting cycle and start burning fat instead of sugar when we enter ketosis, fasting goes way deeper than burning fat and can be considered a long-term sustainable solution to weight management.

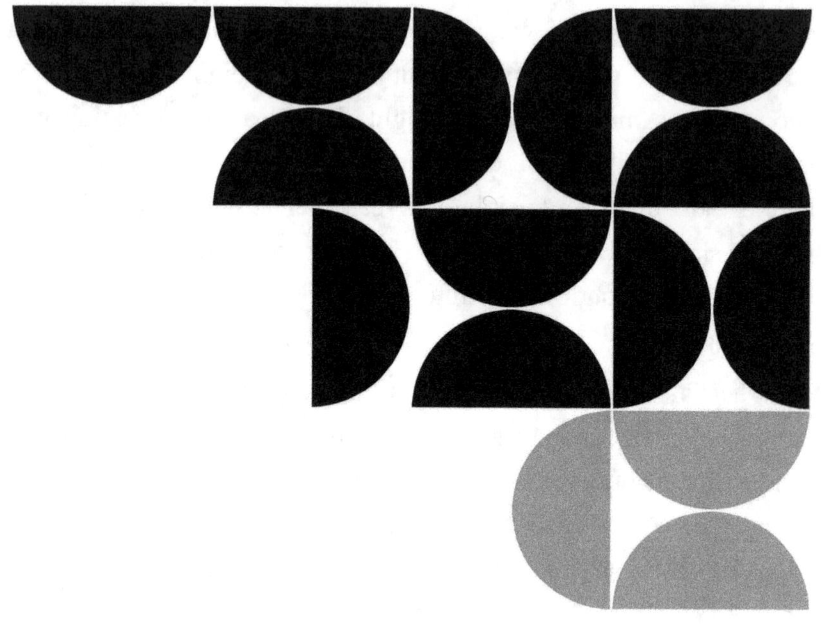

LET'S SHIFT OUR FOCUS TO THE BIGGER PICTURE: HEALTH, NOT JUST WEIGHT LOSS

When we delve into weight loss, it's crucial to remember that it's not the only measure of health. It's not just about shedding excess fat but about overall well-being.

Discussions often revolve around calories and fat burning. If one carries excess weight, the visible fat is just the tip of the iceberg.

Weight gain can stem from various factors, but it's evident that something is amiss.

When we consider fasting as a strategy for weight loss, it's common to think that restricting calorie intake will help us shed pounds. This notion isn't entirely incorrect. During fasting, the body depletes its sugar stores and enters ketosis, burning fat for energy.

However, fasting is not just a tool for weight loss; it's a transformative journey that empowers you to take control of your health. It's a holistic approach that redirects energy from digestion to healing and cleansing. This shift in energy utilization can lead to significant improvements in the functioning of body organs, which may be contributing to the excess weight.

Inflammation is often a significant issue in a body that is not functioning optimally. To protect itself from inflammation, the body's organ tissues retain water. This excess water, along with fat, can contribute to weight gain. However, fasting can help address this issue by reducing inflammation and water retention.

By embracing fasting as a lifestyle, you're not just tackling weight loss; you're addressing the root causes comprehensively. You're triggering ketosis to burn fat, allowing your body to heal, function better, and reduce inflammation. This comprehensive approach to health is what makes fasting so powerful and reassuring in its effectiveness.

Since 2016, I've been on a regular fasting journey. Fasting has not only positively impacted my health but also my looks, despite my age. Instead of focusing on weight loss, I concentrate on health and maximizing the benefits of my fasting sessions. Fasting has given me faith in my body's ability to heal, and one of the positive outcomes of my health-focused fasting journey has been an improvement in my looks.

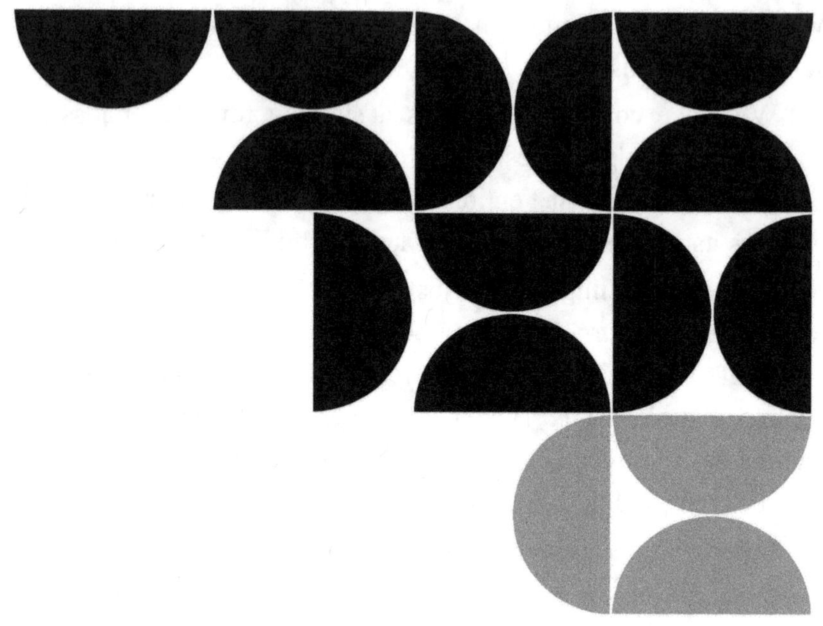

HOW FASTING AFFECTS OUR SLEEP

As with all body functions, fasting will positively affect sleep in the long run. Since I started my fasting journey, I have slept better than I used to. All-nighters are over for me. Since I eat once a day and at night, sometimes this situation makes me go to bed later than I'd like to, but I enjoy not going into a parasympathetic mode during working hours so much that I haven't found the perfect solution when to eat yet.

Fasting will regulate sleep and improve its quality in the long run. It's an entirely different story during the fast, especially with the longer fasts. Since we are not eating, the body finds our bedtime an excellent opportunity to do cleansing, repair, and reconstruction work. This can result in very agitated nights. We are not eating; we are trying to get a good night's sleep, and inside us, fireworks are firing in all directions. This situation is very common. On my longer fasts, it happened to me that I could not get a good night's sleep, but I would nap during the day. The good news is that even with a couple to four hours of sleep, we will feel okay in the morning. Since the body is not busy digesting, reparative sleep will occur in fewer hours.

During those agitated nights, your internal organs may make much noise. There is nothing to be worried about. We should feel good about it. The body finally has an opportunity to do its magical work.

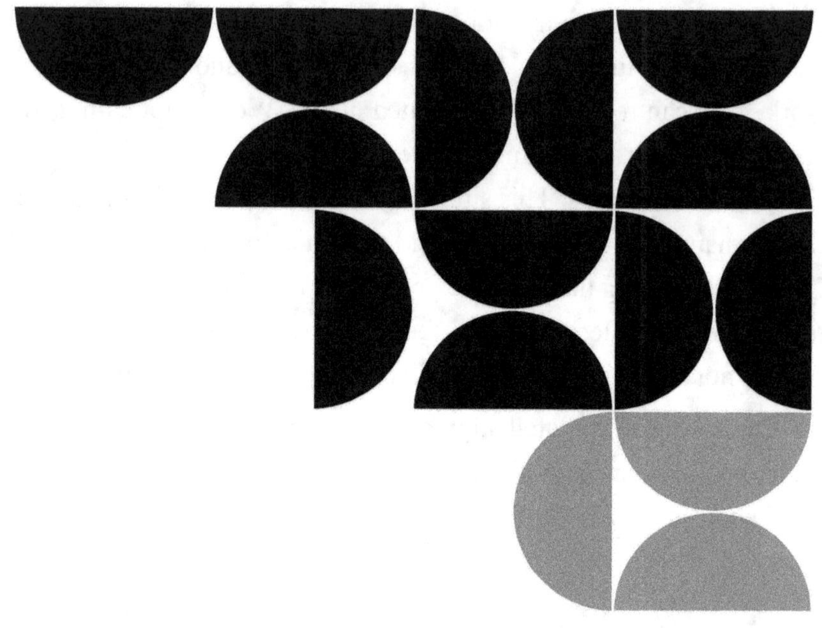

MY UNDERSTANDING OF HYDRATION

One will often hear, "Stay hydrated," especially in the US. When I lived in California, I saw many people walking around with their bottles of water always available. Even though hydration is essential, drinking excessive amounts of water doesn't mean that we are hydrated at a cellular level.

I see the digestive tract from our mouth to our anus as still being outside of the body. Putting something in my mouth, stomach, colon, or anus does not mean that I am putting something inside of my body.

Inside of my body are my blood, my cells. It is one of the reasons why the microbiota of our intestines are so essential. It is the most expansive area of our body that is in contact with the outside world.

For water to enter our cells, several biochemical processes must occur so the hydrating fluid passes the cell's membrane. I personally feel more hydrated if I drink a glass of fresh coconut water, electrolyte water, celery juice, or lemon juice than a half-gallon of plain water. We also need to give our kidneys a break at times. One of the main advantages of dry fasting is that it allows our kidneys to rest and heal.

With dry fasting, I also learned that the body always finds a way to find water. On my 10-day dry fast, even near the end of my long fasting period, I was still producing a glass of urine a day even though I had not consumed any fluids in over a week. Thus, we should not stress out too much about drinking plenty of water but rather focus on having access to quality fluids that will encourage proper hydration.

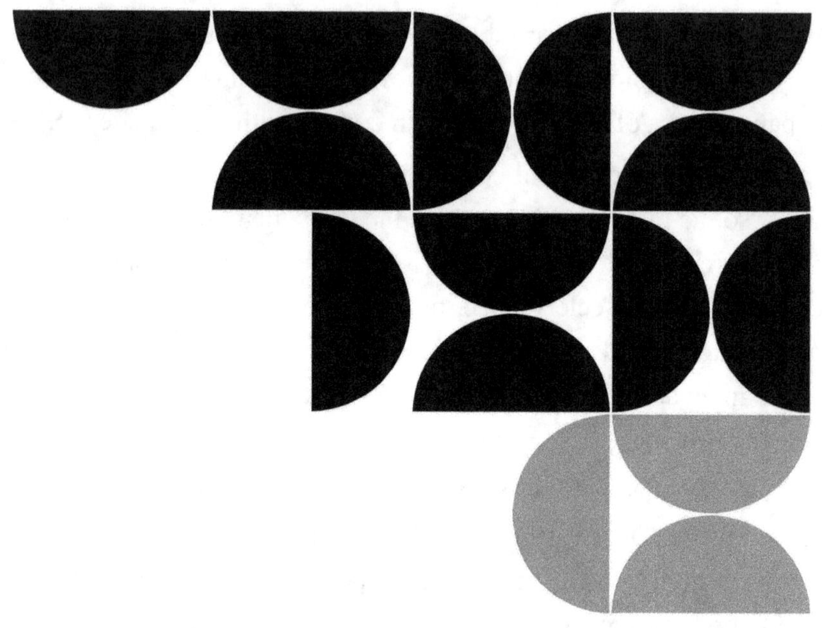

OUR FOUR DIFFERENT ENERGY BANKS

Digestion is one of the most energy-intensive functions of the human body. When we stop eating, that energy is allocated to cognitive, physical activity, cleansing, and repair functions.

Visualize our body's energy allocation during fasting as having four distinct energy banks. Fasting essentially frees up energy from the "digestion bank," allowing it to be utilized for cognitive, physical, cleansing, and repair functions. Taking a cognitive break further boosts our energy reserves for these functions. And when we abstain from physical activity, all our energy is channeled toward cleansing and repair.

Understanding this cascading energy structure is crucial as it effectively empowers us to manage our energy during fasting sessions.

Developing a strong communication channel with our body is key. It guides us on how to navigate our fasting sessions. There are times when we're brimming with energy, engaging in various physical and cognitive activities. Other times, our body signals us to rest, both physically and cognitively.

One thing to keep in mind during detoxification is that a lot of waste matter may be loaded into the lymphatic system, and this can create a strong desire for movement. During my 10-day dry fast, I had abundant energy and walked between 20 to 30 kilometers—12.4 to 24.8 miles a day. It was wild. I would wake up wanting to eat the world and walk through Buenos Aires all day. Even though it was during wintertime, I would do some of my walking shirtless. People around me on the streets were wearing their winter jackets. There were times I had so much energy that I would stop my walk, do some push-ups, and then keep walking.

The point I want to make by sharing this experience is that even the cascading energy distribution structure makes sense, but things with physiology are sometimes complicated. One could try fasting while staying in bed and sleeping the entire time. That way, all the energy would go to cleansing and repair. A situation like this could happen. It happened to me on several occasions that I would sleep long hours during my longer fasts. But keep in mind that movement and getting clean air are also crucial while we are fasting. Once again, the best approach is to listen to our body so we can provide it with the best environment possible to reap the most benefits from our fasting session.

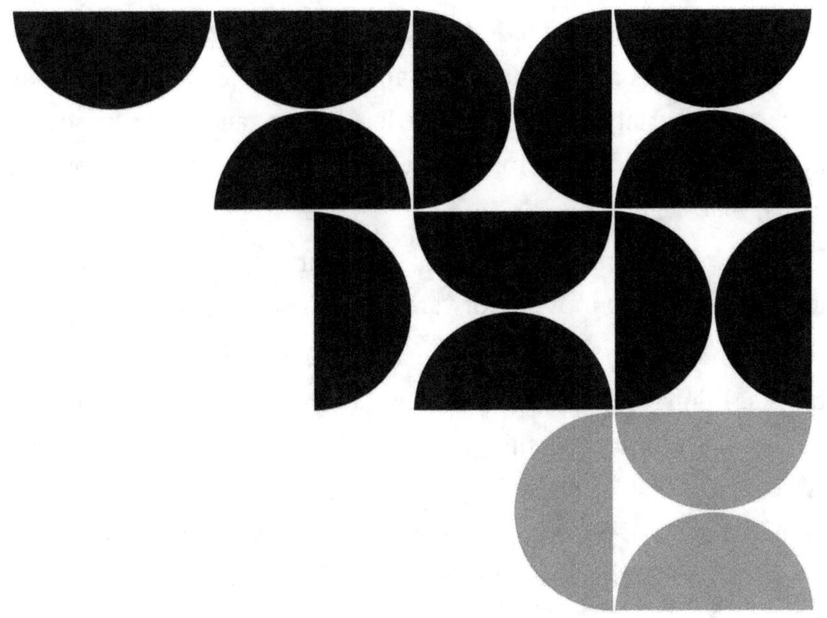

FEELING AND LOOKING YOUNGER WITH FASTING

I started fasting when I was 41 years old. From my mid-thirties to that age, I felt I was getting older yearly. Once I started fasting in 2016, miracles began to happen. I got rid of minor and more severe health issues and started performing better in all areas of my life, which began to make me feel younger every year after 2016.

Don't get me wrong. I am not talking about completely reversing aging and rejuvenating. There are areas where I can observe that I am still getting older, but I perform and feel better in other aspects of life.

Fasting directly and indirectly affects my feeling younger; thanks to fasting, I make better decisions and have learned to use my body better. Rejuvenating, optimizing what I have, and better practices promoting health have brought me to a place where I feel younger every year.

Since fasting regularly puts us on a journey of self-actualization and progress, I am moving forward with everything I do.

Not relating to my chronological age helped me get rid of mental blocks. I don't live my life in relation to my age. For the past eight years, as I am writing this, I've been living as a nomad in Latin America. In 2024, I started my own business, running two different brands. I am still pursuing my rock music career, which I started at 14. I can do it all and have the best life possible at the same time.

Feeling that everything is still possible regardless of our chronological age is a miracle. Fasting is the way!

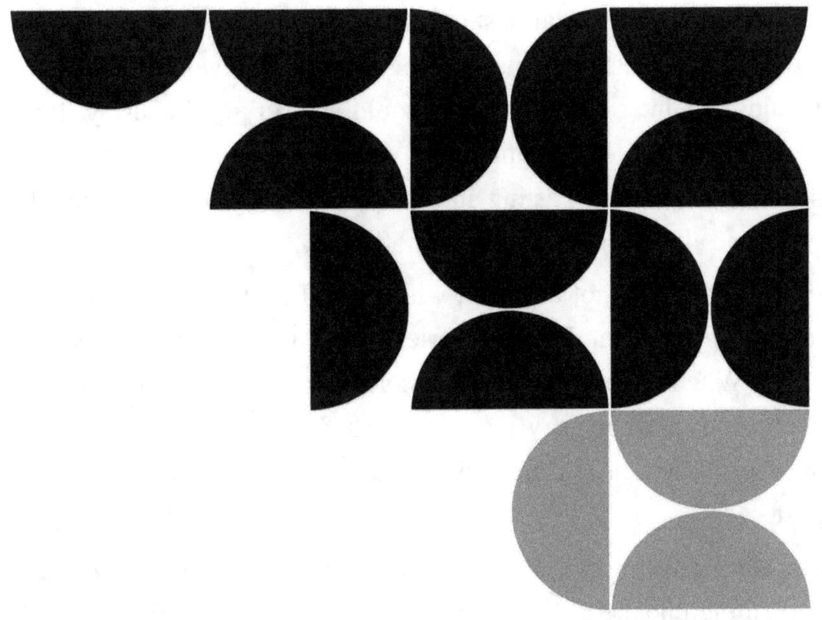

FASTING HELPS ME TO GET CLOSER TO MY TRUE SELF

When I first incorporated fasting into my life in 2016, my only goal was to gain physical health benefits. In the first months of fasting regularly, what was expected happened. I lost weight, eliminated chronic inflammation, eliminated kidney pain, eliminated skin conditions such as eczema and psoriasis, and eliminated hemorrhoids. I also didn't get minor muscular injuries as often.

After noticeable improvements on a physical level, I started to have improved mental clarity and began making better decisions. The unexpected happened almost a year after I got into fasting regularly. I started traveling in time and revisiting my life events. Each time I would encounter past trauma, I would start crying intensely. I had recently moved to Argentina from Europe and was doing the 3/4 - 4/3 fasting pattern. Fasting intensely and being in a new country made me all the more sensitive emotionally.

I am usually not a person who cries. I rapidly noticed that the intense crying that I was experiencing was an emotional healing crisis. When I repeated the time travel to my past, I noticed that an event that made me cry on a previous fast wasn't making me cry anymore. I had healed from that trauma. I could travel more in the past.

After several weeks of intense fasting and eating raw foods, something unexpected happened. All my life goals collapsed. Only my love for making music and my love for the soccer team I root for remained. Until this day, that particular moment of losing all my goals in life was the most difficult challenge that fasting threw at me.

Slowly, I started to recover from it and set new goals that aligned more with the person I was becoming. In reality, I wasn't becoming a new person; instead, I was doing a mental and emotional cleanse, getting rid of all the toxic ideas or negative emotions that were keeping me away from who I was.

With this experience, I learned that fasting cleanses the liver, kidneys, and various other bodily functions, as well as our mental selves, allowing us to get rid of past traumas and ideologies that are not aligned with our true selves.

This experience taught me that we are not only bombarded by pesticides, air pollution, electromagnetic waves, and more but also by ideas that are not ours. These external influences come from our social circles, media, and art. Did you want to become a lawyer, or is this something your family engrained in your brain? Did you want to become a bartender, or was bartending presented to you in a movie as something cool?

In the long term, fasting has allowed me to get closer to my true self and align my values with everything I do. Knowing who I am helps me avoid wasting valuable time and suppress suffering. Each time we do something because an idea is not aligned with what our true self is telling us to do, suffering will result from that action because we are lying to our true selves.

Getting to know my true self and aligning my life accordingly was an unexpected by-product of fasting. What a gift!

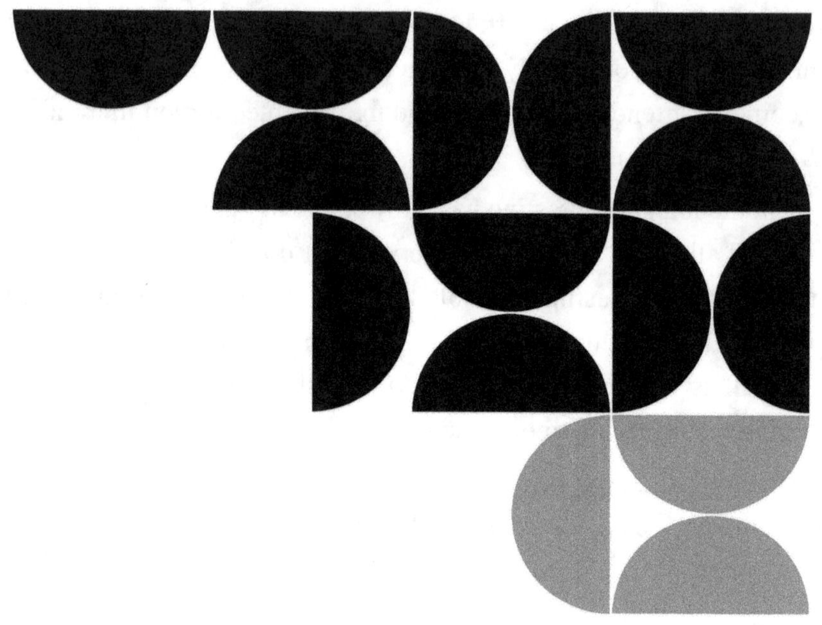

I AM SAVING MONEY FASTING

The last thing I expected when I started my fasting journey was saving money. Depending on how much you include fasting in your lifestyle, it can considerably impact your finances.

I eat once a day. I don't buy breakfast or lunch items. If I skip one meal a day three times a month, that's already a 10% savings on groceries for the entire month; if I skip six meals, that represents 20%.

On the longer fasts of 5, 7, 9, or 10 days, I noticed I wasn't only saving money with food. I realized that so many household items are related to food consumption. I noticed I spent less on soap, trash bags, paper towels, and cleaning supplies. I also noticed that I would save on items like seasonings and oils because I went through them less often.

With the confidence and control over my health that fasting has given me, I have not had health insurance since 2017. It is not something I recommend doing, but it has saved me over 32,000 Swiss francs as I write this in 2024.

With a portion of the money I save on fasting, I am investing it to buy better quality food. I eat fewer meals but of a higher quality. Take someone who eats three meals a day. That will sum up to ninety meals a month. I eat at most thirty meals a month. And if I fast for six days a month, it means I am eating twenty-four meals versus ninety. I do admit that my OMAD will usually have a considerable amount of food since I am only eating once, and I train six times a week. But still, there is a substantial difference.

I go to coffee shops, but I usually don't snack. On rare occasions, if I go to the coffee shop after my OMAD and they have a keto pastry, I may have something to eat. Besides that, I stick to coffee, water, or tea without any sweetener.

What amazes me is that eating about three times fewer meals makes me feel like I am getting all the benefits. I perform better at all levels. Fasting allows me to save money, eat higher-quality food, and feel better overall. With less investment, I get more out of my life. For financial reasons and higher performance, one should absolutely consider fasting.

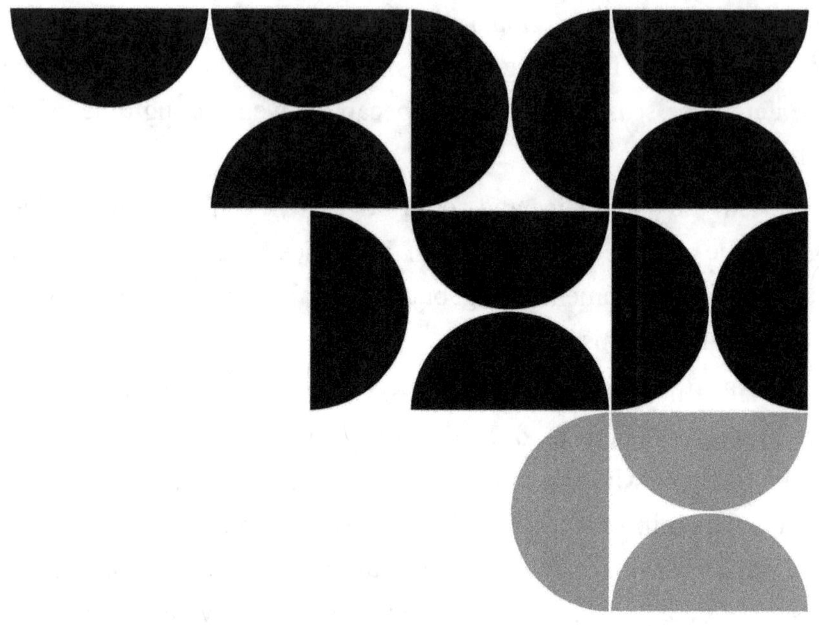

FASTING WITH THE PREPPER MINDSET

Around 2015, I observed that the West was in decline, and the system we were living in might not last for very long. It got me into following seasoned preppers and people predicting the end of Western civilization online. Back then, the dominant idea was to prepare your little bunker in the mountains and stock as much food as possible. I became interested in water, health, food, and energy autonomy. I soon realized that the whole bunker thing in Switzerland was out of my league financially. The price of a simple home starts at one million Swiss Francs in Switzerland, so I needed to adopt a different strategy to prepare myself for the coming difficult times.

If I developed valuable skills, I could join an autonomous community during hard times instead of having my bunker in the Swiss Alps. Soon after, in 2016, I started my fasting journey. I soon realized that fasting was the best tool possible for somebody with a prepper mindset. And the best part was that it was free. A free tool that solves most problems during hard times was a fantastic discovery.

The less is more motto applies to perfection with fasting. I only eat one meal daily and skip 50 to 90 of those single meals yearly. The result is that I am more productive, fit, and happy than when I was eating three meals a day all year round. With all the meals I am saving, one or two more people could afford to live off all that saved food. Stocking food is one thing, but if you can optimize what you have stocked, it's even better,

Fasting taught me how to detach myself from material things. Since I can live without food and water for ten days, not having something to eat does not stress me out. I don't need to run to the supermarket in an emergency situation. I could use those precious moments to leave town or find a solution for survival. Food is not my priority when things start getting rough.

Fasting has strengthened my overall resilience. I am fit and can go days without eating or drinking, which gives me more opportunities to respond to a crisis. I have brought my metabolism to this level without spending a penny.

Besides getting ready on a material level, every prepper should embrace fasting and get prepared from the inside. The stronger your metabolism is, the more resilient you are, and the fewer material goods you need to survive, the more the chances of surviving a big crisis.

Fasting is free and available to everyone. It just takes work, discipline, and dedication.

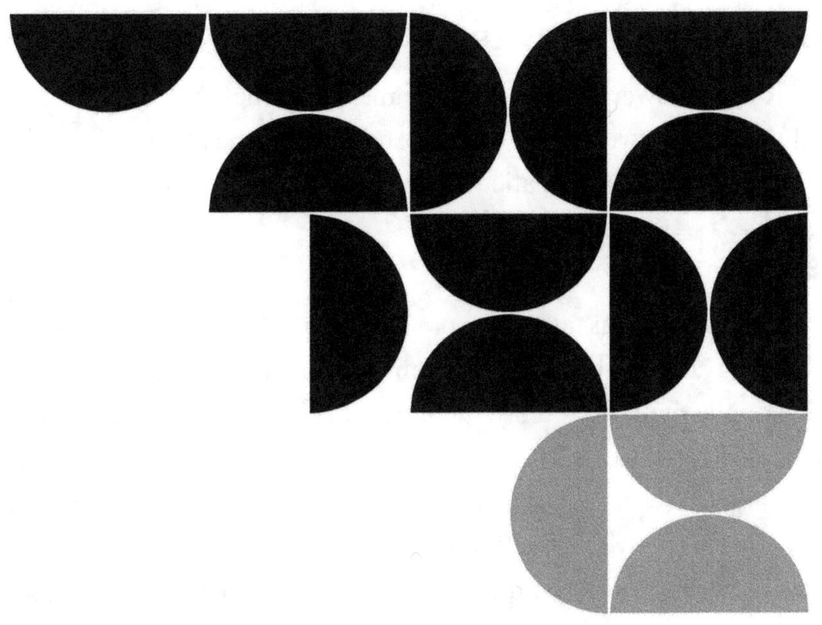

OTHER TOOLS

Fasting is my number one tool for creating the best version of myself, but it is far from the only one.

In conjunction with fasting, I have incorporated other tools and habits into my life, which allow me to progress on this journey.

We can support the functions triggered by fasting to help the body cleanse, move toxic substances, eliminate them, rejuvenate, and feel better overall.

In addition to fasting, here are some of the tools I am using.

COLD AND HOT SHOWERS

Cold showers alone have numerous benefits for the body. Alternating between cold and hot showers can positively affect the movement of the lymphatic fluid inside our bodies.

SAUNA

Sauna sessions also support the lymphatic system, and deep sweating allows the body to eliminate toxins. Overall, it's a very relaxing activity. As I am writing this, I have access to a sauna. I've included going to the sauna six to seven days a week into my routine. So far, the results have been very positive for me. It brings the experience to a whole new dimension. Rather than going to the sauna once a week or a few times a month, going almost every day has given me extra energy, focus, calmness, and overall well-being. In parallel, I've been researching different sauna protocols. It looks like the benefits of going to the sauna are much more numerous than I was aware of. I'll be experimenting more with this fantastic tool.

DRY-BRUSHING

Dry brushing stimulates the lymphatic system and allows lymphatic fluid to move around, especially in the near-surface regions of the body. It also helps get rid of dead skin and eliminate toxins.

KETOGENIC DIET

Reducing sugar and carbohydrates has excellent benefits for the liver and the body. What I love about keto is that it allows me to maintain the mental clarity I acquire during fasting during periods when I am not fasting. I also tend to recuperate faster and need fewer hours of sleep.

EATING RAW

Eating raw can positively affect the body's alkalinization and allow it to absorb more nutrients. When I started my fasting journey, I ate raw for eight months and reaped many benefits.

EXERCISING

I go to the gym five to six times a week. Functional gym, weight training, mobility, cardio, and stretching helped me considerably. I can go to the gym that often per week. Before starting fasting, although I was younger, I could not exercise more than three times a week.

MOVEMENT

Movement is excellent for various bodily functions. I move as much as possible throughout the day and go to the gym most days. Walking, taking the stairs, and movement exercises that can be done anywhere are essential to my daily routine.

SUN BATHS

The sun has become my best friend. Before I started fasting, I would sometimes get sunburns. Now, I expose my skin and eyes to the sun daily. Living in Latin America has helped me a lot by allowing me to sunbathe.

TAPPING MY BODY

Gently tapping my entire body, including my head and face, helps energize me. I start my day tapping my body, moving around, and being in contact with the sun. Taping my body is a part of my morning routine. If it doesn't put me in a socially awkward situation, I will keep tapping my body several times during the day.

GROUNDING

There is actually an entire documentary on this practice. I find it amazing. When I live near the beach, I ground on the sand daily. When I live in a city, finding grounding opportunities becomes more scarce. I find parks; in the worst-case scenario, I go for pieces of grass or dirt on the side of the road. I don't hesitate to take my shoes off and do some grounding. Socially, it can be challenging. At times, people look at me as if I am weird; I've already been mistaken for a homeless person several times when I am shirtless and barefoot. I try to ground myself at least six minutes a day.

BREATHING EXERCISES

This practice is more potent than it seems. When we do it regularly, the benefits augment exponentially.

MEDITATION

As with breathing exercises, meditation has excellent benefits. It's not always easy, but it clears my mind when I can. I am a musician. I also play my instrument freely in a solo jam session to get into a meditative state. Praying also helps me get into a meditative state several times during my waking hours.

SLOW-JUICING

When I first got into fasting, I juiced a lot. I reaped many benefits from it, but I've also made many mistakes since I was juicing many fruits. It's better to have a 90/10 approach and juice primarily vegetables rather than fruits, which are high in sugar. Since I started keto, my relationship with fruits has changed drastically. Although they seem healthy, they can threaten our health if we juice or consume them in excess.

DISCONNECTING

Digital fasting, as I like to call it, helped me immensely. There are days I leave my phone at home and try not to touch any electronic device. It's getting more challenging to do it with my current responsibilities, but it feels incredible each time I can do it. Also, I am organized during the day with my relationship to digital devices and the internet. I don't go on social media first thing in the morning. I don't sleep in the same room where my phone is. I do creative work in the morning, and later on, I do all the communication tasks for my business. At night, I use social media and watch YouTube videos. Getting cheap dopamine first thing in the morning demotivates me for the entire day. I prefer earning my dopamine the hard way by writing, playing music, working on my business, and going to the gym.

WRITING

Writing has many benefits for my professional and personal life. One of them is its therapeutic aspect. Writing empties the mind, helps us organize our thoughts, and records our past experiences. It is the basis for intellectual creativity.

MASSAGES

Massages have multiple benefits. They support fasting and help the body move lymphatic fluid around. One significant advantage of living in Latin America is regular access to affordable, good-quality massages.

MAKING MUSIC

For me, it's making music for you. It can be something else. Making music for me has a therapeutic effect. Through music, I can heal traumas and transform negative energy into something positive and beautiful. It also helps me to release my emotions. When I play the acoustic guitar, touching high-quality wood and feeling the instrument's vibrations makes me feel good.

FACE YOGA

This practice has many benefits. If done regularly, it will directly affect your looks. It is also a spectacular mood lifter. You can type "Face Yoga" in YouTube's search bar, and videos will appear. Some are follow along. I had great results with face yoga and tongue exercises. I also purchased a Jawzrsize device that helps me fortify my jaw muscles and bring more blood to my face. It tends to make me drool, so I find a solution by using it while I shower. The habit-stacking technique in the book *Atomic Habits* inspired me to do so. Since I shower every day, it makes me use the device daily; drooling is less of a problem since I am naked and already wet.

UNDERSTANDING PHYSIOLOGICAL PRINCIPLES

On my longer fasts, I found more time was liberated since I wasn't cooking and eating. To motivate myself to pursue my fasting sessions, I looked for information on fasting. Understanding the physiological principles gives me tremendous willpower to keep fasting. Understanding what is happening inside my body and why I am fasting and going through all this discomfort and challenge is a crucial motivator.

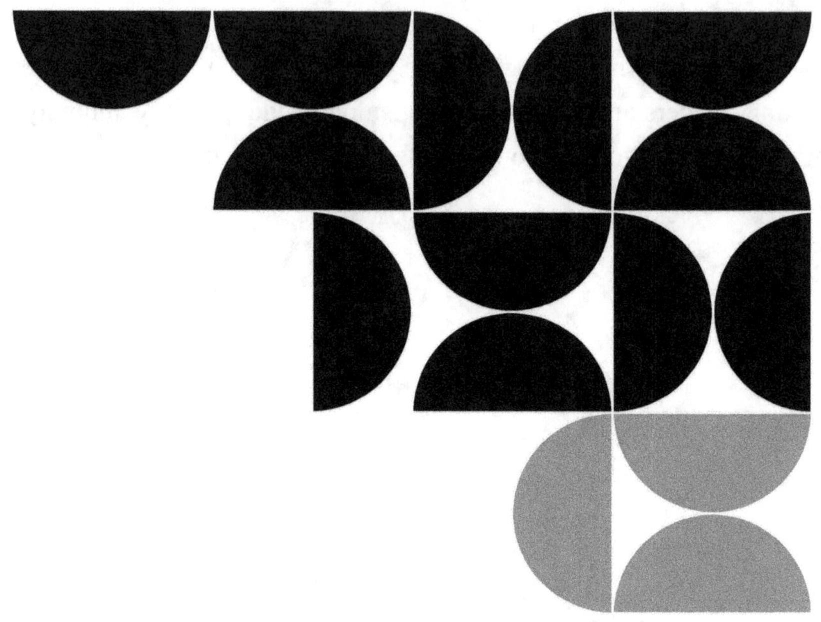

DIFFERENT DIETS I EXPERIENCED

RAW

As soon as I started my fasting experience, I went raw 95% for eight months or so. It was great support for initiating my fasting experience. It helped the cleansing and alkalinization processes. The advantage of going raw is that we keep all the nutrients of the aliments. The challenge is that we must already have an excellent digestive and absorption capacity. If one has inflamed intestines, raw may not be the ideal diet.

NO ANIMAL PRODUCTS

I have done this several times. I usually go for two to three months, after which I hit a plateau. Last time, what made me go out of this diet was that I would eat up to three meals; I would be full but still unsatisfied. I also realized that we eat many carbs when avoiding animal products. The downside of this diet is that it's not sustainable, but I benefited from it temporarily.

FRUGIVORE

Eating only fruits is fun. It has as many benefits as downsides. The frugivore diet makes me consume way too much sugar, and I always had a feeling of never being fully satisfied with this diet. I could never stay on it for more than a week. It's not a sustainable diet for me, but it could have its advantages once in a while. I had a ton of fun going on frugivore diets in places such as Mexico and Peru, where one can find high-quality tropical fruits for an affordable price.

KETO

The ketogenic diet was the most significant discovery for me. Since starting, I haven't quit it. I almost don't eat out anymore, and cooking nearly every day is a significant investment for me, but it has been worth it so far. It is the only diet I haven't reached a plateau on yet. As I am writing this, it has been 16 months that I have been on keto, and it has been great so far.

CARNIVORE

I have yet to explore this diet fully, but since I am on a ketogenic diet, I sometimes tend to go full carnivore, depending on what I am cooking that day. It feels like keto on steroids. It may be the next diet I entirely adopt. It just makes a lot of sense, and I've been reading a lot of positive testimonies.

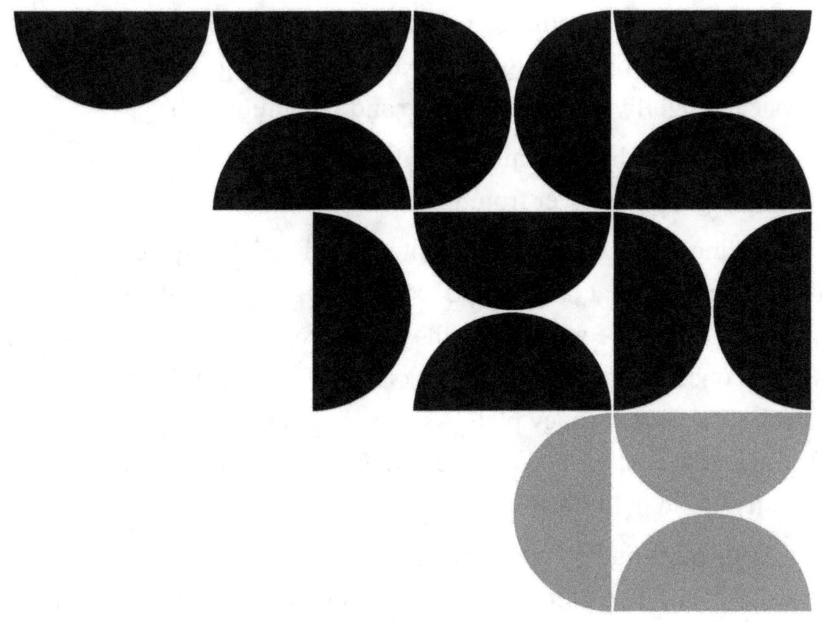

FASTING TO GET BACK ON TRACK

Once we pass the initial stages of fasting and complete a few fasting cycles, we can use fasting as an adaptable emergency weapon, ready for any situation.

If we have had a good run with our routine, productivity, and well-being, we might suddenly feel like we are losing steam. The reasons could be many. In those circumstances, I use fasting to put me back on track. It has never failed. Fasting will tune up our system and eventually put us back on track.

I use fasting to optimize my energy at all levels. Fasting means taking energy from the digestive bank and putting it into the body's physical, cognitive, or maintenance and reparation bank.

Fasting can help us minimize times when we lack momentum and an edge and recover from illness.

Fasting has become my ultimate remedy when I get colds or the flu. I remember that, in the past, when I felt sick, it would at least last a week. During the winter months in Switzerland, I would be in bed at least once a year for a few weeks. Since I've been fasting, I have developed an emergency plan. As soon as I start feeling weak, I start fasting, and I go to bed with a clove of garlic under my tongue. Usually, in 36 hours, I am at 100% again.

With colds and other symptoms that make us feel sick, I noticed that the best thing to do is not to do anything. We tend to find a solution from the outside when we feel ill, but the solution is inside us. No food, no medicine, just a garlic clove, and resting have done mini miracles in my life.

Besides using fasting as an emergency tool against colds, I have noticed that I rarely get sick anymore. Fasting has made my defenses way more potent than they used to be. Getting older, stronger, and more youthful is a great feeling.

To sum up, if we are not happy with how we are feeling or performing, we face challenging symptoms; fasting has been the best emergency tool in my toolbox to get back on track.

Of course, to use it as a tool, we need to integrate it into our arsenal first. Therefore, fasting for the first time when you are sick could have negative consequences if you have never fasted and got a cold. It may be too much for the body to handle at once. Therefore, we should better train ourselves to go through several fasting cycles when we feel good and create an emergency tool with fasting.

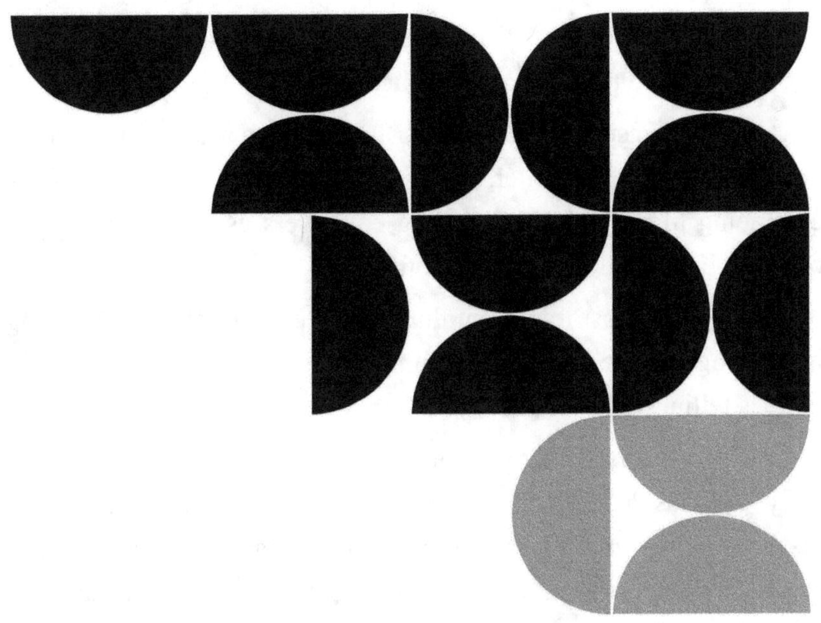

BECOME YOUR FASTING COACH

When we embark on the transformative journey of fasting, different things happen. One of the most important is that the body starts expressing itself. It will express itself through symptoms and how it makes us feel at different moments during our journey, both when fasting and outside of the fasting periods.

The key to mastering fasting and knowing what to do and when to do it lies in our ability to listen and interpret what our body is trying to communicate. Once we master that skill, we can optimize everything in our lives. We will eat the right food and amount at the right time. We will fast the correct number of days when it is needed. We will rest and perform at the right time.

Once we grasp what the body is signaling and act on it, we unlock a world of feeling better, happier, more productive, and fully embracing life. This understanding empowers us to take charge of our well-being and live life to the fullest.

One of the most important things I have learned through fasting is to recognize the true self and unleash its full potential. What the body is telling you is the real you.

We want to avoid getting lost in translation when listening to the body. We must learn to distinguish between what the body wants and needs. Cravings and initial resistance to effort are not what the body needs. We need to learn how to differentiate between those three states through experience.

If we crave ice cream with lots of processed sugar, it is not our body communicating what it needs. An underlying issue manifests as a craving—the same as resistance to a challenge. We take an ice bath, go to the gym, go out for a run, start a fast, and all those things. Once we are about to get started, resistance will emerge.

So, how do we decode these signals? My approach is to respond to the signal and observe how the outcome makes me feel. I've learned the hard way that indulging in sugary ice cream or junk food doesn't lead to long-term well-being. No addiction is sustainable. Similarly, I know that swimming in Lake Geneva during winter will be a challenge, but the post-experience will be invigorating. We need to experiment with the body's signals in the same way.

Now, I have done so many fasting sessions that my body requires me to fast when I go without fasting for a while. My body will tell me if I need to go on a short tune-up fast or a longer one. Even with my daily intermittent fasting, my body will tell me whether the fast should be dry. Sometimes, when I do my 18 hours of intermittent fasting, my body will tell me to go on for a couple more hours.

To summarize, to understand what our body is trying to communicate, we need to start fasting so that the body gets into the habit of expressing itself. Imagine a conversation between two people, and only one is always speaking. The second person will never have the opportunity to express herself. This is exactly what's going on when we eat three meals a day and snack in between. We are suppressing the body's ability to express itself. The same goes when we constantly numb the brain with TV sound. We don't allow our thoughts to emerge.

It's crucial to interpret the messages our body sends and act on them. Through trial and error, we'll gradually decipher what our body is trying to communicate. Once we understand and act on the message correctly, we'll gain momentum, reinforcing the positive cycle of health and well-being.

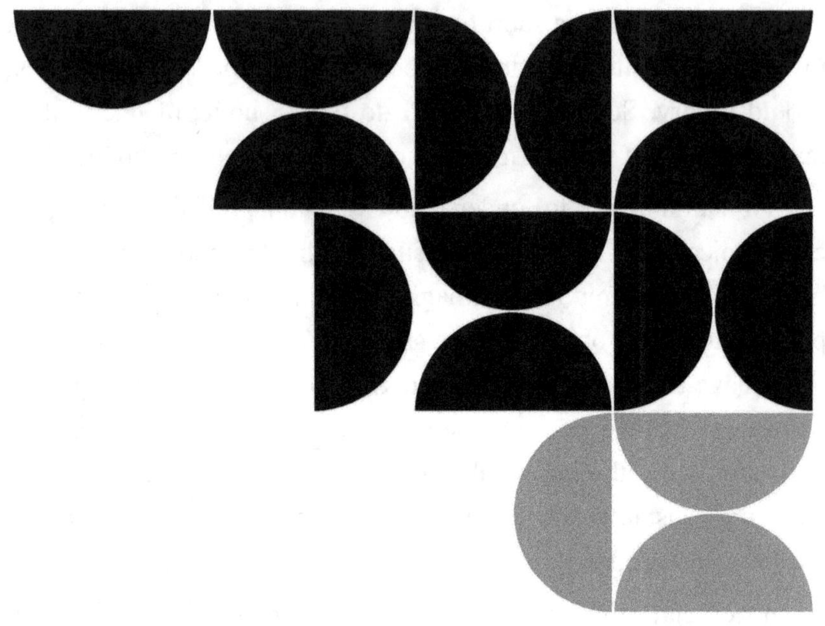

FASTING HAS BECOME
MY GUIDE IN LIFE

Once we start fasting regularly, the body begins expressing itself through symptoms and how it makes us feel.

Suppose we focus on what the body is trying to express and act upon it. In that case, we start making decisions that allow the body to do its job in better conditions, and we make progress toward having a better functioning body and mind.

Once we master listening to and understanding the messages our body sends, we can distinguish between what the body wants and does not want.

After fasting for many years, my capacity to smell what is contained in the air has improved tremendously. I can smell cigarette smoke from several feet away. When the neighbors are cleaning their apartment, I can smell the type of cleaning product they are using. Not only can I smell the scent, but at the same time, I receive a message from the body telling me if the smell is good or bad for me. That way, I can avoid toxic environments and try to find and enjoy places with clean air.

I have developed a similar detection mechanism with people; it is as if I can sense very quickly if the person is toxic or if it is a person who is going to bring something positive to my life. Since I have been almost in total control of my social life for the past few years, I avoid toxic people at all costs, and I can do that because I am capable of understanding the message my body is sending me.

When I must make macro-level decisions, I communicate similarly with my body. I can listen to my true self and make the best decision. In this situation, I almost bypass my brain for decision-making. I focus on my body's gut and heart region and try to feel what I want.

If I have a big decision to make and can't decide, I specifically use fasting as a decision-making tool. I start a fasting session that lasts several days and then reflect on the decision I have to make. Disconnecting from material needs allows me to get closer to my true self and make a decision aligned with where I genuinely want to go in life.

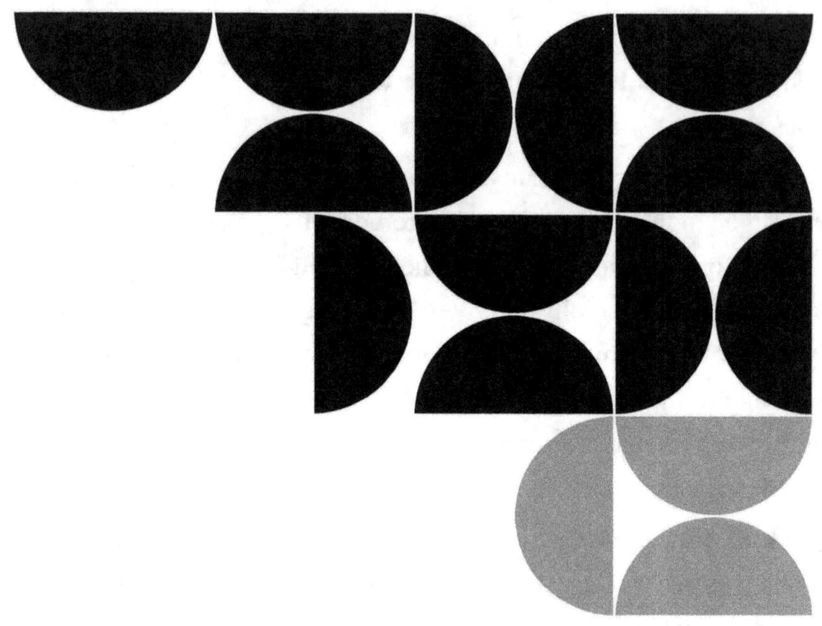

WITH FASTING, I DON'T NEED A MEDICAL DIAGNOSTIC

It's a radical notion to suggest that we can trust our bodies to self-regulate without needing constant medical diagnostics. Our bodies are remarkably self-aware, knowing what's happening and what needs to be addressed. Our bodies maintain a to-do list of malfunctioning organs and systems. They only ask that we give them the space and time to heal.

I stopped trying to be the CEO of my health and turned myself into an angel investor. I give my body a capital of fasting days, and my body does the rest. I give my body the best fasting environment, incorporating techniques and healthy behaviors to go in and out of fasting, and my body gets the job done.

My priorities might not be aligned with my body's priorities. I may suffer from back pain on the right side, and relieving pain may be my priority. My back pain problem may come from a liver-related problem. So it can be that the body needs to fix the issue with the liver before my back pain is fixed.

Since I trust fasting and my body more than doctors, I stopped going to them. For an emergency mechanical problem like a broken arm, of course, I am going to seek medical help. I still go to the dentist, but my body is the best doctor for everything else. Since I know my body is on top of things and knows what needs to be fixed, I don't need to know what's wrong with me. Instead, I will focus on doing my part of allowing my body to fast, exercise, eat healthily, meditate, do breathing exercises, go to the sauna, and so on. I am responsible for providing the best conditions for my body to heal.

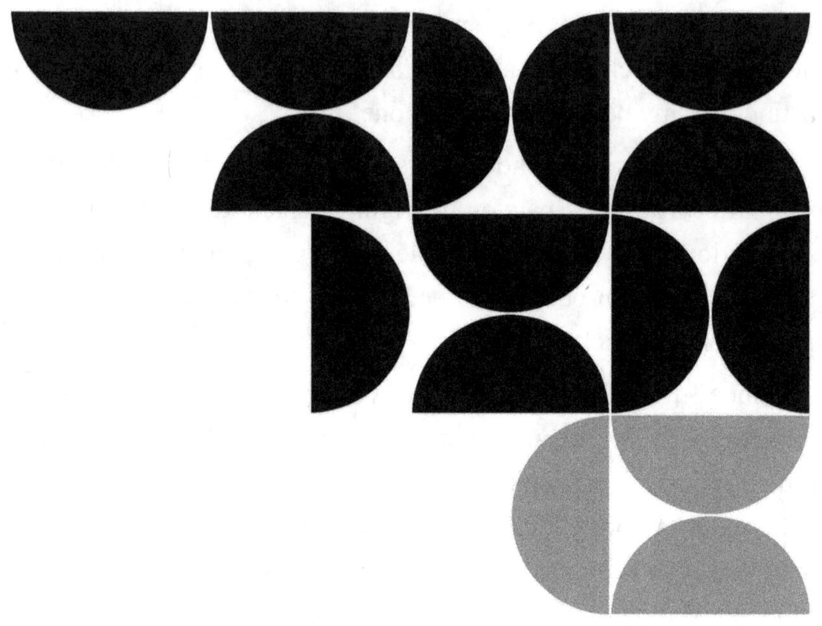

FASTING PATTERNS

Fasting is like going to the gym. It's a practice that needs to be incorporated into our routine and practiced regularly to see results.

There is no single formula for fasting. To see improvement, we need to increase the number of fasting hours and embrace a strategic approach.

Just like with exercise, we tend to plateau after a while if we always do the same exercises. Similarly, fasting is crucial to challenging our bodies in different ways. This is where the concept of fasting patterns becomes significant. We can see more effective results and maintain our body's adaptability by varying our fasting hours.

As we embark on our fasting journey, we may need to be more expansive in various fasting patterns due to our low fasting capacity. However, from the very beginning, we have the power to build fasting patterns that align with our current level. This personalization and control over our fasting journey can be empowering and encouraging.

For example:

Say we have a fasting capacity of 10 hours of fasting a day. With that fasting capital, we can build a weekly fasting pattern. We could fast 10 hours a day, three days a week, challenge the body with two days of fasting 12 hours, and not think about fasting the remaining two days. Congratulations, we have a weekly pattern. We can execute this pattern and see what happens. After a couple of weeks of implementing this pattern, we could pass to three days of fasting, 12 hours, two days of 10 hours, and a couple of days of rest from fasting, and so on.

As our fasting capacity grows, we will have more options to create elaborate and challenging fasting patterns.

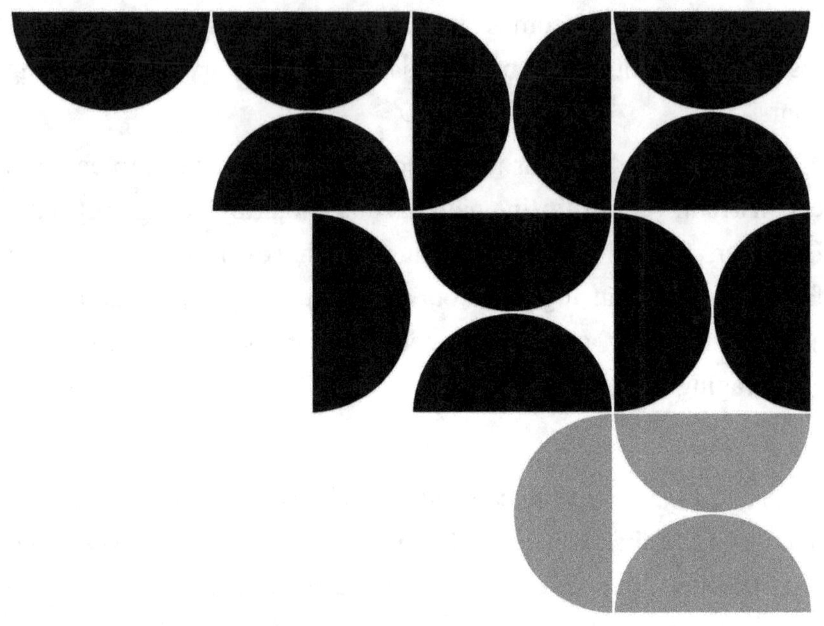

HOW TO BUILD FASTING PATTERNS

My strategy for building fasting patterns is akin to playing a video game. It's about setting challenges, leveling up, and gaining new skills. This approach not only makes fasting more engaging but also helps to improve fasting and adaptation capacity.

I intend to incorporate challenging fasting periods to improve my fasting and adaptation capacity. Fasting longer and more frequently will give me more building blocks to create new and more challenging fasting patterns.

Consider this fasting pattern: We fast for 36 hours, have an eating window of 6 hours, fast for another 36 hours, and break our fast. This pattern requires us to be able to fast for 36 hours, which is the initial step toward achieving a higher level of fasting. Once we accomplish this, we have a new "building block" to incorporate into our weekly pattern.

A pattern I often execute consists of intermittently fasting six days a week with an 18/6. One day, usually during the weekend, I skip the only meal and go for 36 to 42 hours of fasting. Sometimes, I do it twice weekly: 18/6 for five days and skip two meals. The only requirement to execute this pattern is to be able to fast for 36 to 42 hours.

Therefore, the key to successful fasting is to construct "building blocks" and then experiment with these blocks to create new fasting patterns. For instance, we can try the 3/4, 4/3 weekly fasting patterns, which involve fasting for 72 hours (3 days) and then intermittent fasting for the remaining four days of the week. The next week, we can fast for 96 hours (4 days) and then intermittent fast for three. This pattern requires us to first build our capacity to fast for 96 hours. Once we achieve that, we can implement the 3/4 4/3 fasting pattern.

To sum up, we first need to fast long enough to create a fasting building block. Once that building block is under our belt, meaning we can fast that long without feeling challenged, we can then start constructing patterns made with that fasting block and periods when we allow food intake.

Why even bother with patterns?

To get the best out of our fasting journey and keep moving forward, we must constantly challenge the body in different ways so we don't hit a plateau. With fasting, yes, we need discipline, and yes, we need routines, but we have to be very careful so that routine does not put us to sleep, so to speak. Switching fasting patterns is a great approach to challenge our bodies from different angles. That way, our metabolism and adaptative capacity will strengthen.

Fasting patterns stimulate not only the body but also the mind. They push us to be creative. Experimenting with different fasting patterns gets me very excited. Fasting patterns are one of the elements of fasting that made me so passionate about fasting. I am a musician, and I actually find some similarities between fasting patterns and time signatures in music.

When we zoom out and think about fasting at a macro level, we can conclude that it is not dieting or calorie restriction. Fasting is the process of timing our food intake. It's a binary system: ON/OFF. Fasting patterns are the organization of those ON/OFF moments at a more elaborate level. Fasting is mastering the timing of food intake to heal and optimize our bodies, mental health, and spirituality.

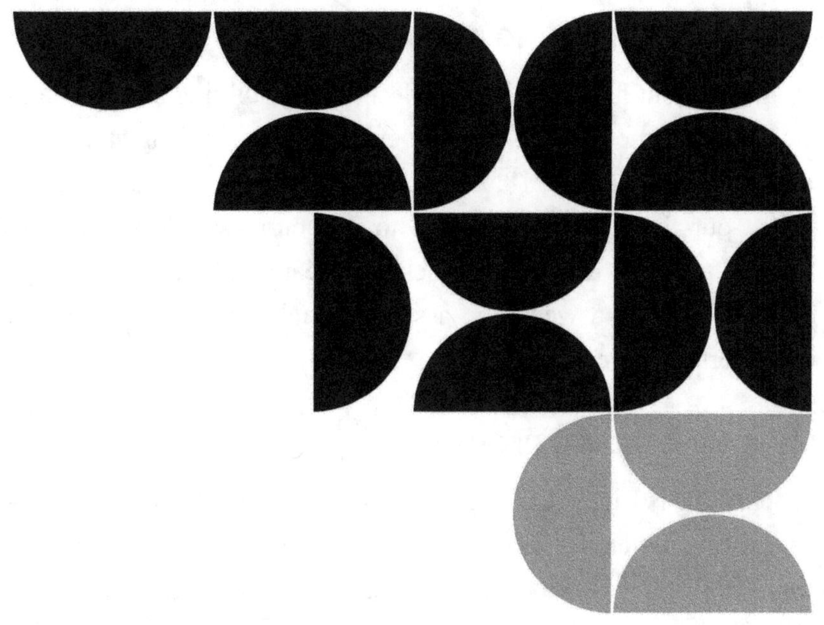

BUILDING BLOCKS FOR FASTING PATTERNS

To build fasting patterns, we need to develop fasting blocks first. I mean a defined number of fasting hours during which we are comfortable. If a block is still too challenging to complete, incorporating it into a pattern will be even more difficult, so it is crucial to have those blocks under our belts before building patterns.

INTERMITTENT FASTING BUILDING BLOCK

Intermittent fasting is our smallest fasting building block. The 8-hour one is something that almost everyone does during sleep. We can build 10, 12, 14, 16, 18, 20, and 22-hour blocks from there. Once we get our fasting capacity to 18 to 22 hours, we already have a versatile toolbox of building blocks to create patterns. Then, it's a matter of picking a week and assigning each day a building block with a certain logic behind it.

24-HOUR BUILDING BLOCK

This one is tricky. Our intuition could make us think that the 24-hour fasting pattern is pervasive, but I avoid it in patterns. Here is the reason why. Since a day on Planet Earth is 24 hours, if we fast 24 hours, then we take at least an hour or two to eat, then if we try to fast another 24 hours the next day, we will start drifting from the Earth's chronological rhythm. Fasting for 22 hours and eating for two would work. Even fasting for 23 hours and eating for one hour will allow us to repeat the pattern daily if needed. In brief, the 24-hour building block will create a problem if we want to repeat it daily. But it is doable as a stand-alone fasting period.

THE 36–42-HOUR BUILDING BLOCK

I use this building block a lot in my fasting patterns. I only eat one meal a day. Once in a while, I skip that meal and go for a 36–42-hour fast. The 36 hours here is the minimum. The number 42 comes from observation. On average, my one-meal skipping fasts last that long. As long as we stay under 48 hours, we can break that fast between 36 and 47 hours. I enjoy that flexibility. It allows me sometimes to eat my OMAD earlier than usual. I also use this pattern if friends invite me for breakfast or brunch. Instead of refusing a social invitation, I say, "Okay, I'll see you for breakfast," but I don't eat the day before and break my fast with them earlier that day.

THE 72-HOUR BUILDING BLOCK

After 36 hours of fasting, we enter ketosis. At 48 hours, autophagy and rejuvenation of mitochondria begin. By 72 hours, the body resets its pallet, making us less reliant on salt and sweets for pleasure. This potential for health benefits can be a motivating factor for those considering the 72-hour fasting block. I even heard one testimony on YouTube that a patient with type 2 diabetes was able to cure his condition by dry fasting for 72 hours. My experience and intuition tell me that completing a 72-hour fast once in a while will reset certain body functions. I've done it many times on my journey as a part of a pattern or stand-alone.

96-HOUR BUILDING BLOCK

At the 4-day mark, we are starting to get into prolonged fasts. These can be used as a building block of a pattern or as a stand-alone 96-hour fast.

5-DAY BUILDING BLOCK

The 5-day mark is when we enter deep fasting. If we dry fast for that long, we will experience exciting mental experiences.

6-DAY BUILDING BLOCK

When I reached step 7, I did a 6-day fast as part of the stairs pattern. This pattern could be integrated into weekly patterns. We can imagine fasting for six days, eating for one, and fasting for six days.

A WEEKLONG PROLONGED FAST

I did several 1-week fasts. One was during the last step of my seven-step stairs fast. A fast that long is pretty advanced. It took me over a year and a half to get to that level. Fasting for a week has a psychological effect, too. It feels like we went on vacation for a week and we came back home.

9-DAY PROLONGED FAST

I've completed two as stand-alone fasts, but they can be incorporated into patterns. After breaking a prolonged fast, returning to our comfort zone, fasting a day or two a few days after our long fast has some benefits.

10-DAY PROLONGED FAST

In 2018, I did a 10-day dry fast. I initially wanted to go for 12 days but reached my limit on day 10 and decided to break it. I haven't felt the need to fast that long since.

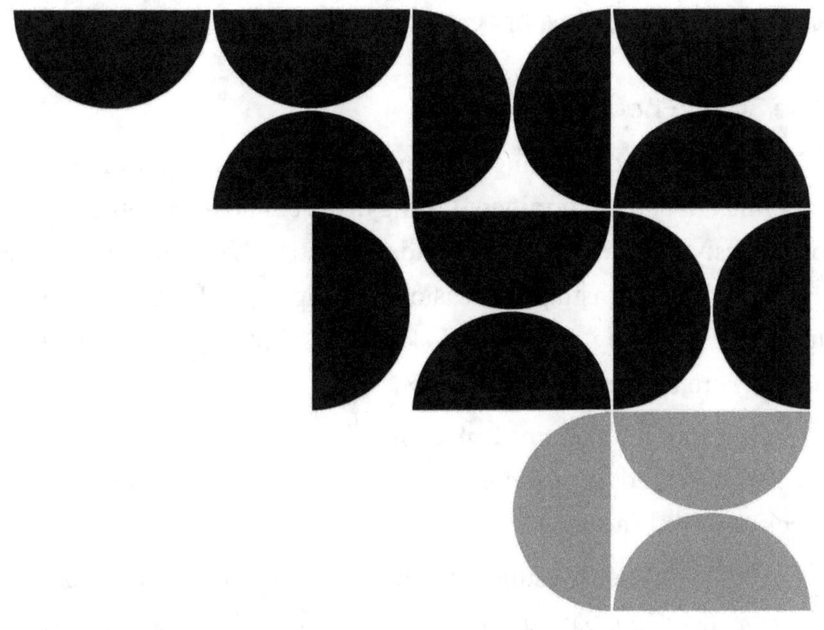

A LIST OF DIFFERENT FASTING PATTERNS I HAVE EXPERIMENTED WITH

Building fasting patterns and experimenting with them is one of my favorite aspects of fasting. As I challenge my body differently, thinking of new patterns stimulates me mentally.

WEEKLY FASTING PATTERNS FOR INTERMITTENT FASTING

The 36–42-hour fasting

The 36–42-hour fasting pattern is the one I use most often. My baseline is a daily intermittent fasting of 18/6. I do it so naturally and effortlessly that I don't even consider it fasting. With that routine of 18/6 intermittent fasting, I occasionally skip my only meal and wait until the next day. This meal-skipping situation makes me fast somewhere between 36 to 42 hours.

To create the pattern, I place it into the week. In 2018, for 56 weeks, I skipped my meal every Sunday. I sometimes skip twice a week or as little as once a month.

The 36–42-hour fasting acts like a tune-up of my metabolism. When I do it on Saturdays or Sundays, I tend to start the week refreshed. Doing it twice a week allows me not to feel as tired near the end of the week. When I skip my only meal of the day, I tend to go to bed earlier and usually wake up more refreshed and well-rested than the days I eat.

The 3/4 - 4/3 Pattern

This one is already advanced. It consists of dividing the week into three days and four days. We fast for three days in the first week and eat for four. The following week, we fast for four days and eat for three. We keep going this way for several weeks.

The 1/1 Pattern

This one is straightforward and may seem easy initially, but it is one of the patterns that challenged me the most on my fasting journey. It consists of eating regularly for one day, not eating the following day, and doing it as long as possible. On the first day of fasting, the body goes into fasting. When we break our fast, regardless of length, the body adapts to returning to its comfort zone. Doing the 1/1 pattern puts us in a constant situation of adaptation. We are constantly either going into fasting or coming out of it. Both have their challenges for the body. Therefore, even though this fasting pattern seemed easy at first, it was one of the most challenging ones I have experienced.

The Stairs Pattern

This is a pretty advanced and involved pattern. One may need to make time for it. Fitting it into a working routine may be challenging, but with prior training, it is not impossible.

The Stairs pattern consists of fasting one day, eating one, fasting two days, eating two, then three, then four, etc. Once we complete the fifth step, the entire fast equals 30 days. I did one of the five steps and one of seven. Both have been very beneficial for me.

The logic behind this fast is to challenge the body and then rest for an equal time of the fast. The fasting pattern of the stairs is built on the principle of hormesis.

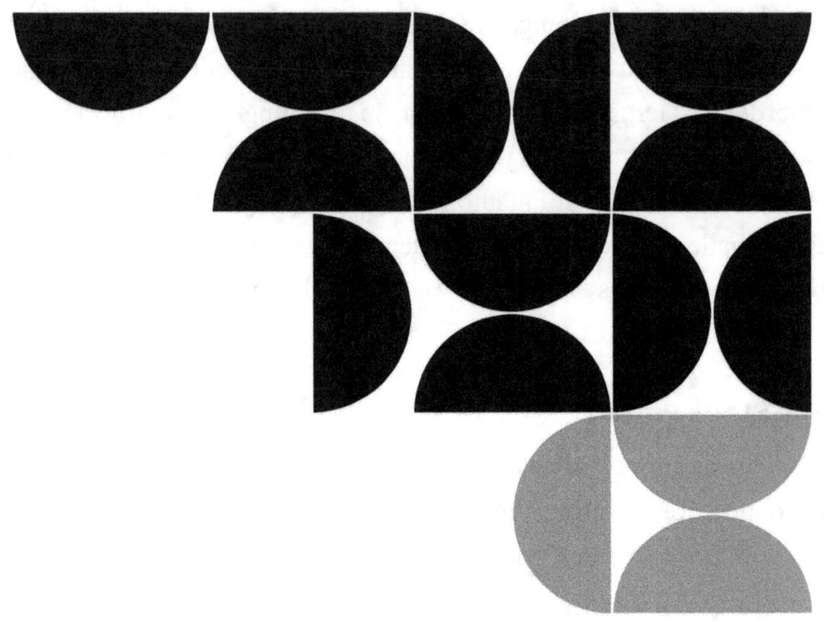

FASTING AND KETOGENIC DIET

I started fasting in 2016. The 18/6 intermittent fasting has become my baseline. I almost forgot what breakfast or lunch was after a while. I've done numerous fasts, going from 36 hours to 10 days. I have mostly been dry fasting until recently.

In March 2023, I discovered the ketogenic diet. I am writing this in June 2024. Besides four cheat meals, I've been on the ketogenic diet since I embraced it.

The ketogenic diet was the missing piece of the puzzle for constantly feeling fabulous. During my fasting periods, I'd elevate my consciousness and have enjoyable mental clarity, but as soon as I broke my fast, the magic of fasting would disappear. It was highly frustrating. I'd be productive, creative, and inspired during the fast, and as soon as I broke it, I would feel like a lesser version of myself.

Keto allowed me to retain some of the mental magic of fasting even when not fasting. It has been a life changer. I sleep fewer hours and recover like I was sleeping longer. I have good mental clarity even when I am not fasting. My digestion improved. I go to the bathroom more regularly, and the consistency of my stools is soft but compact. It has become effortless to clean myself after going to the bathroom.

The ketogenic diet forces the body to burn fat instead of sugar for energy. I already knew that the body was going into ketosis after the 36 hours of fasting. With the ketogenic diet, although we are eating, we keep the state of ketosis, which turns our metabolism into a fat-burning machine. The results have been spectacular for me. The combination of fasting regularly and when we are eating, adopting a ketogenic diet has been my winning combo. I have 15 months of experience writing this with keto and fasting combined, and I've been more energized, productive, and happy than ever.

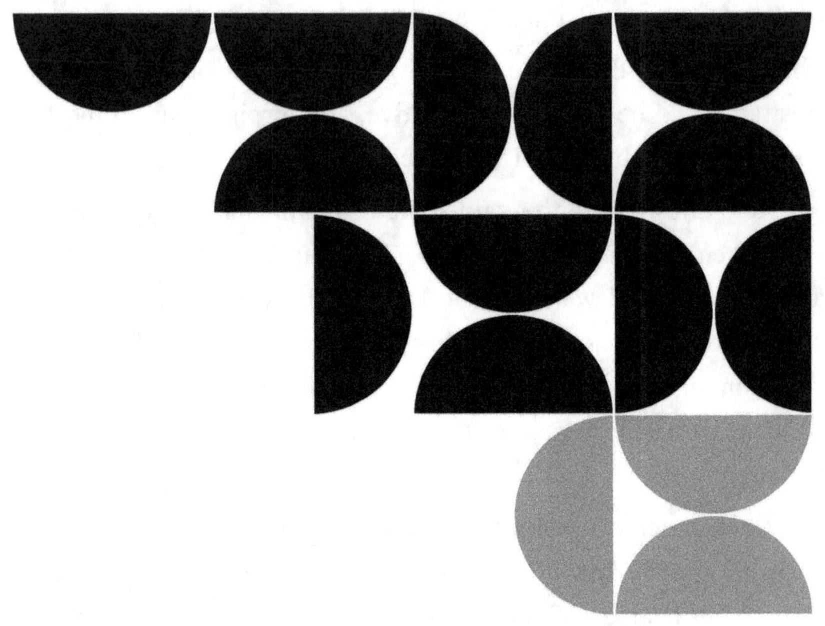

KIDNEY FILTRATION

Discovering kidney filtration was a big step in my journey to 100% health. Around June 2017, I had already been practicing fasting for over a year, and I suddenly found out about kidney filtration while doing research online. When I say kidney filtration, I am not referring to the kidneys filtering blood but rather to the kidneys expulsing waste matter through urine.

The kidneys are one of the exit points for the waste matter that the body produces while cleansing. It is essential to know if our kidneys are filtering or not. We can find this out by monitoring our urine. We will have to pee into a transparent jar. If we can see through the jar and the urine, the kidneys are not filtering. If the urine is opaque and we cannot see through, it means that the kidneys are filtering and the body is getting rid of waste matter through the kidneys.

When I first started to monitor my urine, even though I had been fasting regularly and mainly eating raw for over a year, I noticed that my kidneys weren't filtering. I researched more and learned about all the factors that favor kidney filtration. Dry fasting, eating astringent fruits, dry brushing, hot and cold showers, and hot compresses are all factors that promote kidney filtration. I did them all except for the hot compresses directly on the kidneys. I went to the pharmacy and bought one of those gel packs that can be used cold or hot.

I put the gel pack into boiling water, and when it was almost burning hot, I wrapped it in a T-shirt and placed the hot pack between my back, on the level of my kidneys, and the bed where I was lying facing the ceiling. After several sessions of applying the hot compresses, my kidneys started to filter. My urine was finally opaque, full of waste matter. If I put the jar filled with urine to rest, after 25 minutes, the waste matter in the urine would pile up at the bottom of the jar. It looked like snowflakes.

After filtering the waste matter through my kidneys, I immediately felt better. It was a fantastic feeling. It was as if I had been wearing an old-school all-metal diving suit all my life, and finally, I could take it off. My body started to feel more flexible, and I had better energy. Still, to this day, the day I made kidney filtration work for me is one of the most important milestones on my fasting journey.

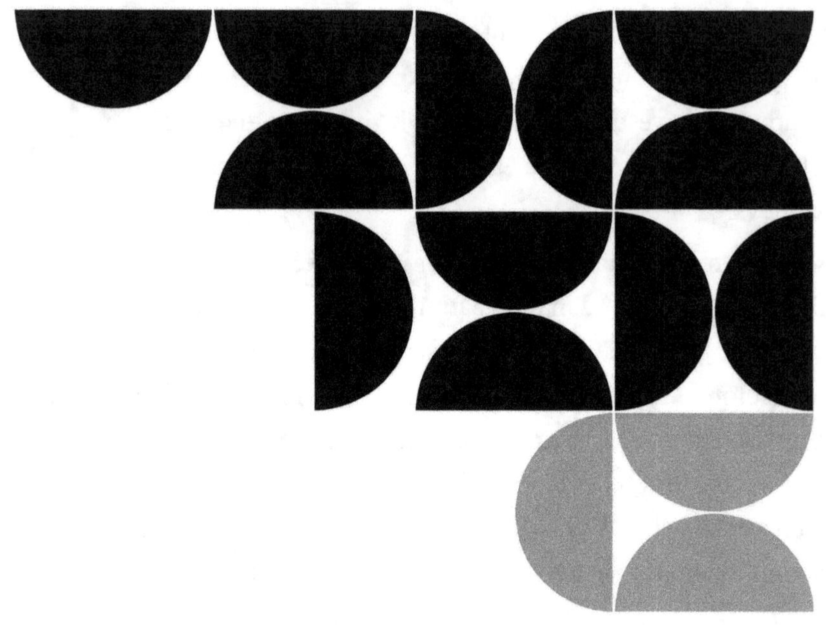

FEELING RESISTANCE AND MAKING PROGRESS

Once I initiated my fasting journey, some of the results were immediate. However, one general pattern I've noticed is that overall progress comes in stages. For example, if I were filling a pool with water with my fasting work, the water would cascade into a bigger pool once I filled the entire pool. Each time I cascaded to a new pool, it felt like reaching a higher stage of a video game.

Usually, before cascading to a larger pool occurs, the last moments of being in the current pool feel laborious, as if fasting is presenting me with some resistance. On the other hand, once I pass to the next pool, I feel like I have accomplished something big, and now that struggle is behind me, and new challenges are ahead.

My observations may sound abstract. The idea I want to convey is that the body is doing its repair and cleansing work, which probably consists of a group of subtasks. Once the task is completed, the body can use that improved function and focus on a different repair and cleansing process set.

During our fasting journey, we will face periods of resistance and quasi-plateauing, which can be challenging and tedious. We must remember that we are very close to getting promoted in our fasting journey, and things will get much better and more exciting very soon.

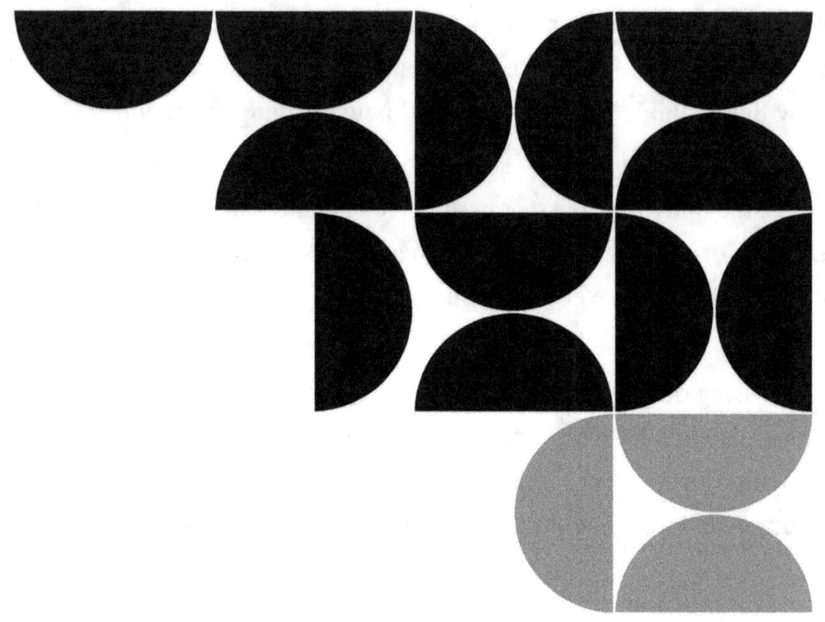

I DON'T BELIEVE IN DISEASE

Since I have adopted fasting as a lifestyle, I don't believe in the concept of disease anymore. I learned to embrace the symptoms as my body's expressions. The body always functions how it should. The body is like a calculator that always gives us the correct output, even when someone suffers from an advanced imbalance in health condition. If we enter 4+4 into a calculator, it will always give us 8.

We can act at the input level. We can control the environment to a certain extent, and we can control the input regarding nutrition, social interaction, emotions, and healthy practices. We need to input positive things if we don't want to be in the red with the calculator output. The advanced imbalance in health conditions can be broken down to the input. Of course, genetics are also part of the input, but a series of negative inputs brought the body to output after the equal sign to an advanced imbalance in health condition.

Modern medicine with physiological issues tends to make the symptoms disappear rather than the cause effects. By going the contemporary medicine route, we not only don't cure the problem at its roots, but we also destroy the message the body is trying to send us. In addition, we get the side effects from medication. The whole cocktail makes us lose ground. The entire thing becomes a driving experience on an icy road. We are sliding on one side of the road, trying to stabilize the vehicle by turning the wheel to the opposite, sliding to the other, and so on.

It took me almost a year after starting my fasting experience to quit medication. It is one of the best things I have done for my health. As I write this, I haven't used medicines except for local anesthesia when I go to the dentist. Life without medication has been working exceptionally well for me.

Rather than believing in disease, I prefer to believe in equilibrium. When the body's equilibrium is lost, symptoms will appear. It is our responsibility, then, to bring the body back to its equilibrium. Therefore, I am all for the acceptance of symptoms. I see how the body makes us feel daily, as small messages and symptoms as strong messages.

I also don't believe that we catch a disease. "I was walking on the street, and I caught cancer." It just does not make sense to me. Cancer is a condition and not a disease, even with viral ones. I don't think that when we encounter viruses, if our equilibrium is substantial, the virus will do anything to us.

During the so-called pandemic period in 2020, I was unable to leave Uruguay for the first six months. I did not experience any symptoms. Back then, I thought it was because we were secluded as a country, and the fact that they closed the borders may have helped. Once I left the country in September 2020, I kept traveling. I refused to put a mask on unless it was mandatory and I could get in trouble. I took the bus, the plane, the boat. I traveled all across Mexico and Guatemala. I did not experience any adverse symptoms.

My immune system was strong enough. I was regularly fasting, and I had faith that nothing would happen to me because I was fasting periodically, which made me feel strong. I also believed that COVID-19 was just a flu-like virus pumped up with media propaganda. All these factors made it so that COVID-19 did not exist for me.

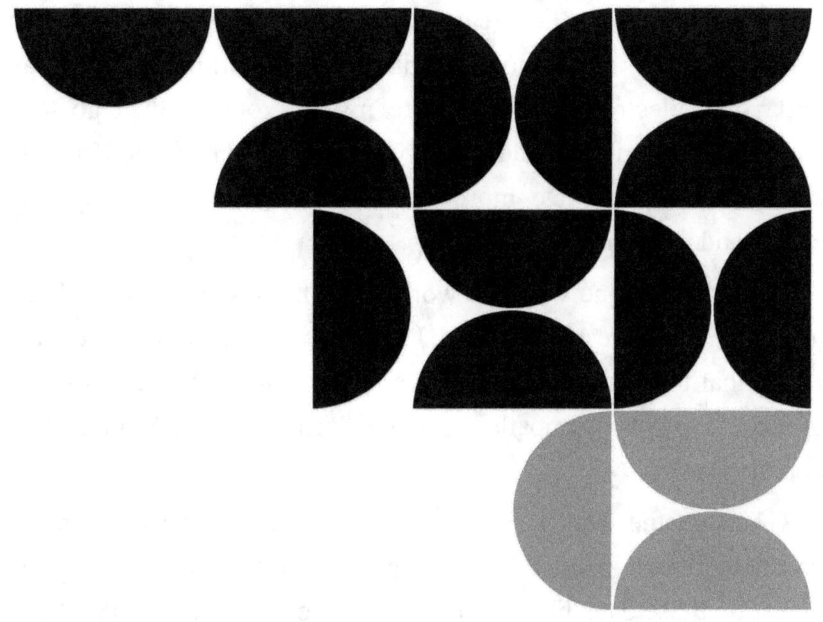

FASTING INCREASED MY PRODUCTIVITY

After passing the initial stages of adaptation to fasting, my baseline has become one meal a day and intermittent fasting of 18/6 hours. In addition to that, I skip my only meal a day between 50 and 90 times a year. I don't eat for two to three months every year.

When I wake up, I get sunlight and fresh air, tap my body, stretch, and jump around. I then pray and start working. Food is not a distraction in those early hours, a fact that can lead to magical moments of creativity and productivity.

Since I am on the ketogenic diet, my body is burning fat; I don't get any cravings throughout the day. I keep working. I'll have an unflavored electrolyte drink before my workouts. I then go to a coworking or digital nomad-friendly coffee shop with a good internet connection to complete more work. I'll only consume sugarless coffee and water at the coffee shop.

Once I am done with my work day, I'll cook my keto OMAD, have dinner, and rest a bit. Then, I'll work more before going to bed. I love that food is not distracting me during the day, and I don't go into a sleepy parasympathetic mode during the more productive hours.

Usually, the days I skip my OMAD are magical in terms of productivity and inspiration. Not having to buy groceries, cook, and digest on those days liberates about three to four hours, where I can work, play music, and walk. The following mornings or days when I don't eat, I usually wake up earlier than when I eat and am full of energy. It gives me very productive mornings and high energy throughout the day. I typically look forward to breaking my 36–42-hour fast, which makes the day go by very fast.

Fasting has been a productivity booster for me. I have more time to do the things that matter and more energy and focus.

Snacking isn't incompatible with fasting. If, for instance, you do an 18/6 intermittent fasting, you can snack during the six-hour eating window. The important part is not to eat during the 18-hour window.

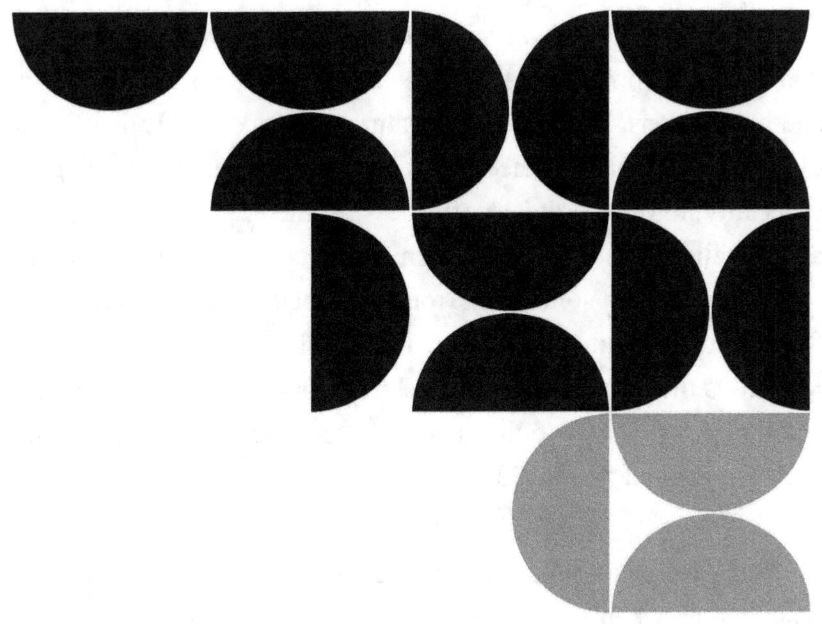

FASTING WHILE TRAVELLING

Fasting while traveling is a tool I developed throughout my years as a nomad. We must remember that fasting while traveling is a pretty advanced way of fasting. Traveling by itself will stress our organisms, so when we add fasting to the travel, we add extra stress to our metabolism.

Fasting while traveling does not have extra benefits in cleansing and reconstructing the body. It might even be the opposite. That said, naturally, I leaned toward fasting while I traveled; since I travel a lot, it has become a habit.

I found the following advantages to fasting while traveling: I don't need to worry about finding healthy, affordable food at airports and bus stations. I can go to the bathroom less often. It may sound like a small detail, but since I travel with my guitar and music gear, especially in Mexico, it isn't effortless for me to go to the bathroom at bus stations. They have an automated rotating door system where one needs to insert some coins, rotate the metal structure, and access the bathroom. With all my gear, I don't fit into the allowed space. Mexico is the last place I would ask someone to keep an eye on my belongings while I go to the bathroom, especially in the north of the country. For that reason alone, fasting while traveling has helped me a lot.

Not having to think about eating and drinking makes traveling easier. Also, when I arrive at my destination, I go straight to bed if it's already late. Since I haven't eaten, I tend to rest better. It's always a great pleasure to discover a new place with the mental clarity that fasting provides and slowly set a routine with healthy habits in my new destination.

Not having to spend money on food is a big plus while traveling. Since I started eating keto, I've been cooking a lot at home. I must control the salts, oils, and overall produce I use. In general, but especially in airports and bus stations, restaurants are mostly there to make money. They are not there to build a community and provide the best quality food to the people.

Fasting while traveling makes the experience go smoother and faster for me. I often find a spot in the waiting areas to play my guitar. I will use my laptop offline to write; on the plane, it is usually a surprise to people when they see me refusing the complimentary food and snacks offered. It is often a profound moment for me that while fasting, I observe people accepting all the low-quality food being offered, including all the processed snacks and soda. The paper cups are coated with gluten-based chemicals for hot beverages. After people have finished eating, I observe the quantity of trash produced with a single meal when the flight attendants pass through the aisle to recuperate the garbage.

It makes me think we have a long way to go as a society to become healthy again. It seems as if everything is designed to kill us slowly in modern society.

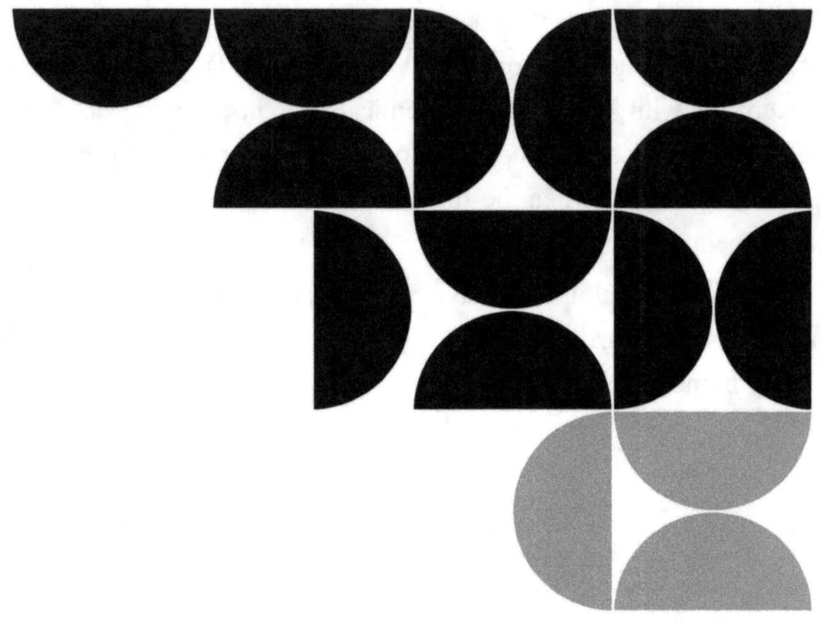

MY THREE-STORY PYRAMID OF WORK

In my last 9 to 5 job, several colleagues of mine experienced burnout. Although work challenged me, I was fortunate not to experience such a fate. After losing my job and starting my fasting journey, I felt constantly better than the weeks before. It was an ongoing experience of feeling always better than before. After a year of making progress, I came to the following conclusion. If I have been feeling better every day for the past year, I must not have been feeling that well before. I was doing fine while working my 9 to 5, but I was probably very close to being burnt out, too. Losing my job probably saved me. It was a saved-by-the-gong type of situation.

I decided to change my approach to work. I needed to generate money, pursue my musical endeavors, and stay healthy, so I divided work into those three categories. I realized I needed to be healthy to accomplish money-generating work, produce music, and perform live shows in the four corners of the globe, living as a nomad.

The basis and first story of my work pyramid is health. I consider fasting, going to the gym, cooking my meals, meditating, going to the sauna, getting massages, walking, grounding, etc., work. The vast majority of the things I share with you in this book constitute the basis of my work pyramid.

I have all my income-generating activities on the second story of the pyramid.

I have placed work related to creativity and my contribution to culture on the top and third pyramid stories: music production, writing books and articles, playing live shows, and traveling the world. This third story would only be sustainable with the two below.

The eureka moment for me was when I started taking practices related to health as seriously as I take conventional work; everything fell into place. If I am dry brushing, going to the gym, or having a sauna session, I don't see those activities as leisure time but as work and an investment in my future. That approach got rid of all sentiments of guilt.

There have been days that I will work six to seven hours only on health. Nobody will pay me directly for that work, but deep inside, I know it's my primary moneymaker. Not only will I have a return on investment when working on the other two layers of the pyramid, but I will also get more out of life because I am doing this work.

How can I make time for it? First, I live a solitary and nomadic life. Secondly, I was able to escape the 9 to 5 hell. Freelancing gave me more flexibility initially, but I needed more. As a solopreneur, I have better control of my time. Since work does not feel like work, I see all three layers of the pyramid as work that is easy to accomplish for me. I wake up and work on all areas. I even see cooking my meals as work; one way to look at it is that I work 16 hours daily. The other way to look at it is that I hacked my brain by perceiving work as fun and leisurely. Now, all my waking hours are lots of fun and promote self-actualization.

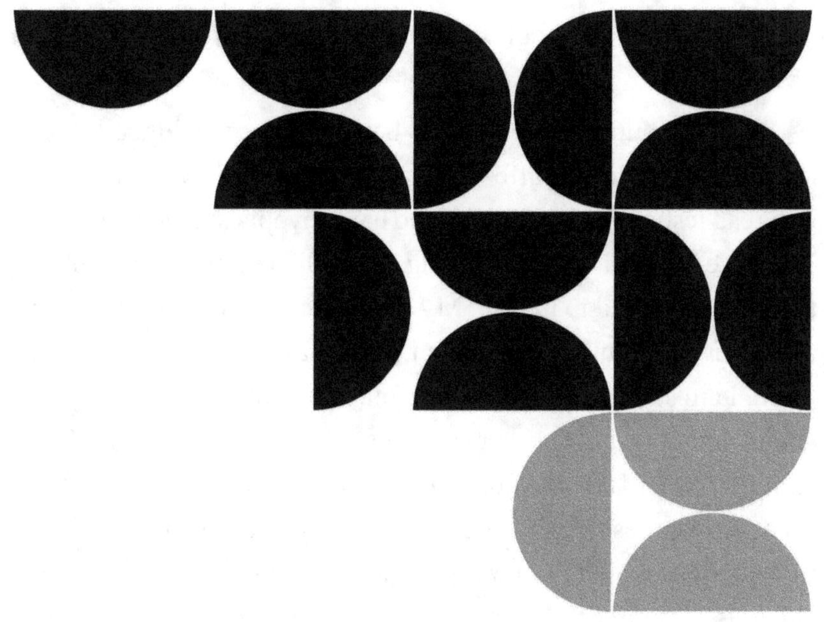

IF WE ARE NOT 100% HEALTHY, WE MUST KEEP WORKING

Feeling okay and doing okay is not acceptable. If we are not 100% healthy, we must keep working on our health. I've been regularly fasting and doing activities to support my health since 2016. Am I 100% healthy? The answer is no. I did tremendously improve my health condition and got rid of many symptoms along the way, but I still have a long way to go.

We must realize that as we work toward health, many negative factors are still attacking us from all sides. To make progress, we need to work hard enough to outweigh the negative effects of our environment.

Why do I think I am not 100% healthy? Since childhood, I have had impaired vision. I suffer from astigmatism and hypermetropia. I have read testimonies of people who have myopia and who were able to achieve 20/20 vision with fasting. With all the fasts I've completed, it has not happened to me yet. My vision would improve a bit during my longer fasts, but in the long run, I may have even lost some of my vision. I am still spending way too much time on screens. My vision would probably be far worse without me fasting, but here's the reality. I am not 100% healthy. I have also experienced slow hair loss since my twenties. Ideally, if everything were working perfectly well in my body, I would not be experiencing hair loss. I have gray hair, which is a sign of demineralization. I am constantly trying to remineralize my body, but for now, I can't say that I have reversed anything.

So, when I look at things from this angle, even though I have accomplished a lot in improving my health, I still have a long way to go. That is why, once in a while, we must see the glass half empty to realize that we need to take even greater measures and work harder on our health to get the results. 100% health is not a miracle. It is the minimum we should demand from life. We live in a sick society, which makes the 100% health idea belong to the realm of miracles. It should not be this way. 100% health is the minimum requirement we should have for life. We are not on this planet to be unhealthy. We all have a mission that we need to accomplish. We have no time to waste with health issues. We should always strive for 100% health. If we are not there yet, we can keep working until we meet the minimum requirements, which is 100% health.

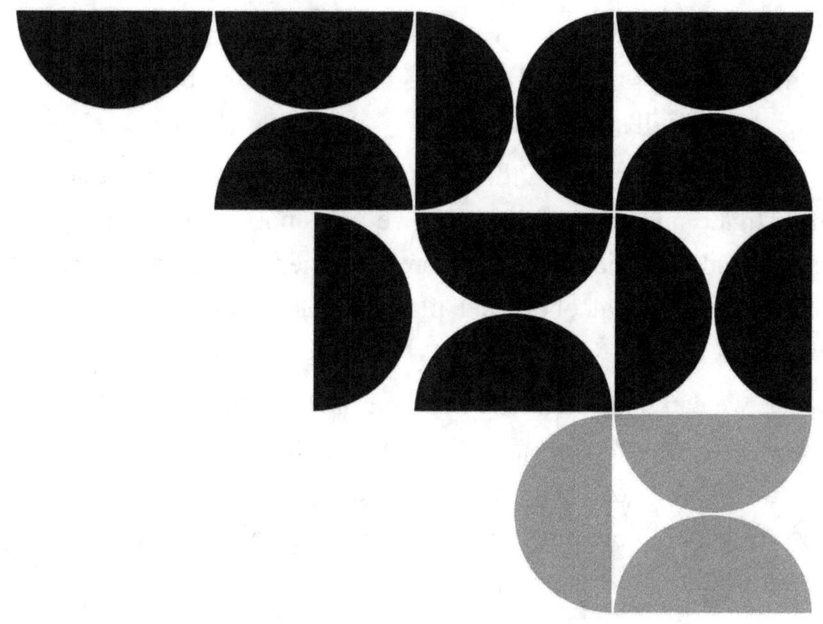

BEFORE QUITTING AN ADDICTION, REPLACING IT WITH A SUSTAINABLE HABIT FIRST

My take on addictions is that they exist for a reason and fulfill a function within the human machinery. Imagine an old bridge or a building that is in terrible shape. Neither of them could stand on their own. To prevent them from collapsing, the municipality where they belong has built supporting structures around the buildings to keep them standing. I'm sure you've seen crutch-type structures before to keep falling apart buildings still standing tall. I see addictions the same way as those crutches that keep buildings in lousy shape still standing.

That's why before quitting any bad habit or addiction, we should investigate and think about why we are smoking, watching porn, eating junk food, doom scrolling on social media, binge-watching TV shows, drinking alcohol, and playing video games for extended periods.

If we can understand the function the addiction is fulfilling, we can devise a sustainable alternative and replace the bad habit before quitting it for good. An analogy to the physical world would be restoring an old building or bridge before removing the crutch-type structures.

In my personal experience, I got rid of several addictions. One thing that surprised me was quitting drinking coffee for six straight years. The surprising aspect of quitting coffee was that I did not try to stop. At the same time as starting my fasting journey, I got into the habit of slow juicing daily. Before starting my fasting journey, I was heavily addicted to caffeine. I was the type of person who would say, "Please do not talk to me before I drink my first coffee in the morning." The sad part is that during my 9 to 5 job, I would drink between 8 to 10 cups a day to feel okay and keep functioning intellectually.

As I started to juice, I went from eight to five and then three cups of coffee a day without even noticing it. I only drank one cup a day once I moved to Buenos Aires in 2017. I then quit coffee altogether until recently. Now, I consume coffee in moderation. I had gone to Buenos Aires to open a third-generation coffee shop that would only use plant milk. Quitting drinking coffee made me quit the coffee shop project as well.

Once I analyzed why I had a caffeine addiction, I concluded that I was probably demineralized, and most likely, my adrenal glands were underperforming. Caffeine gave me a short-lived energy boost, but it wasn't sustainable and was tiring my adrenal glands even more. With juicing, without knowing it, I found a sustainable alternative to coffee. I was able to remineralize my body and regenerate my adrenal glands. It is why I naturally cut down on coffee effortlessly.

With this logic in mind, we can analyze why we are addicted to certain things. Why are we smoking? We could get the same relaxation and mental clarity results with breathing exercises. Why are we getting cheap dopamine with social media first thing in the morning? We may need to learn how to earn our dopamine the hard way. We may be trying to fill a social void with social media. Seeing friends in the real world and socializing with strangers could help us reduce the time spent on social media.

Once we understand the function our addiction is fulfilling, we can look for sustainable alternatives and include the alternative in our lives without quitting the bad habit. If our analysis and replacement are correct, the bad habit or addiction will go away effortlessly.

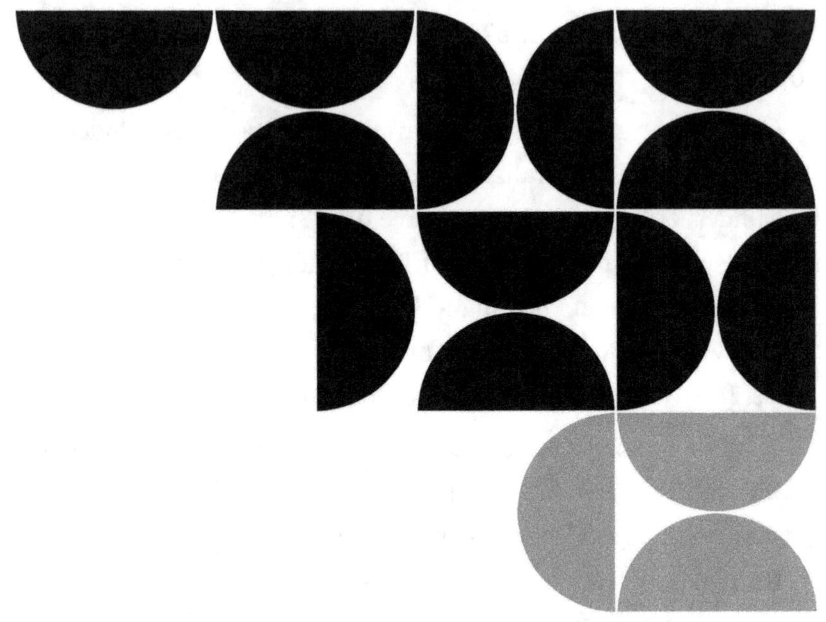

THE MAGICAL EFFECTS OF FASTING

So far, my fasting experience has been incredibly transformative. I see it as a miracle of life. During my social interactions, when the topic of the conversation is fasting, I find myself trying to convey the idea of a miracle. I cannot always express it well enough so that people understand why I am so amazed by fasting.

In this chapter, I will explain where the magic of fasting happens with precise observations. Nothing I will convey has a scientific basis; I am only conveying my observations.

THE POSITIVE DOMINO EFFECT:

To me, the body has a to-do list of repair and cleansing tasks it has to perform. When fasting allows the body to execute such tasks, the body starts executing them. From my experience, those tasks come in groups, and when the groups of tasks are completed, we graduate from our current level of well-being to the next. The domino effect starts when a task or group of tasks about a specific organ or function of the body is repaired, enhanced, or tuned up, and it will positively affect other organs and functions of the body.

Let's imagine that after completing one or several fasts, the body had on its to-list to fix certain liver functions. Once those tasks are completed, and we break our fast and return to our comfort zone, we have a better functioning liver. A better functioning liver will positively impact other organs and functions of the body, which will function better and affect further organs and functions they directly associate with. It is where the magic comes in. All of a sudden, a positive domino or butterfly effect takes place. This is why, after longer fasts, we can still observe improvements in our health and well-being weeks after completing a fast.

I see fasting as investing; in this case, it feels like investing and getting compound interest in return.

THE RIGHT ACTION, THE RIGHT TIME, THE RIGHT AMOUNT:

Another circumstance where I observe the magic of fasting is when we act perfectly with our body's communication. Once we get good enough at deciphering what the body is communicating to us and have enough experience to respond with the right action at the right moment with the right amount, the body improves its performance at all levels. This situation also results in an upward spiral-like dynamic. Everything starts functioning better if we interpret the body's message correctly. The right amount of food, sleep, and rest allows the body to do that activity at the proper time.

Little decisions we make throughout the day can have significant positive consequences. We go to bed at the right time, eat the right amount, and exercise where the body is challenged enough. Fasting the exact amount of time the body needs at that very moment is a fine-tuning action that can have amazing effects.

Fasting has so much to offer and acts at so many levels. When we start fasting regularly, we experience exponential improvement in our well-being.

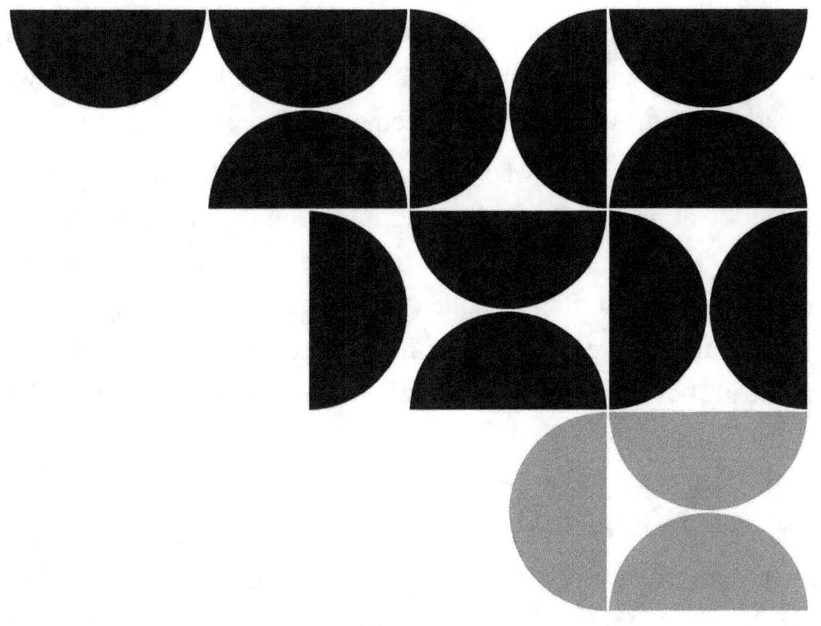

FINDING OUR TRUE PURPOSE IN LIFE

Fasting taught me what was good for my body and what was not. Something similar happened with thoughts and with being able to make better decisions. I started avoiding thoughts that weren't constructive. Then, I tried to answer deep existential questions such as:

- What am I doing on this planet?
- What is my true purpose in life?

The answer to these questions can be continuously redefined. I am not talking about constantly changing direction in life, but as we experience things, our purpose becomes more precise.

If you are at a place where you cannot answer that question at all, I have great news for you. Finding our true purpose is an exciting journey. I firmly believe each of us—every individual human, animal, fish, insect, flower, pollen, etc.—has a purpose in this world. As humans, we are blessed with high consciousness. We can think and learn new skills and languages, making our adventure on this planet fascinating.

Fasting is an excellent tool if one has yet to learn one's purpose. It is a great way to get to know who we are and what we want and don't want. In addition to fasting, I suggest traveling as much as possible and trying as many different activities as possible. Eventually, we will find passion and our true purpose in life. Learning new languages is also a game changer in experiencing life and seeing things differently.

If you have already found your purpose in life, fasting will allow you to focus better on your goals, be more efficient, and avoid wasting time on health-related issues.

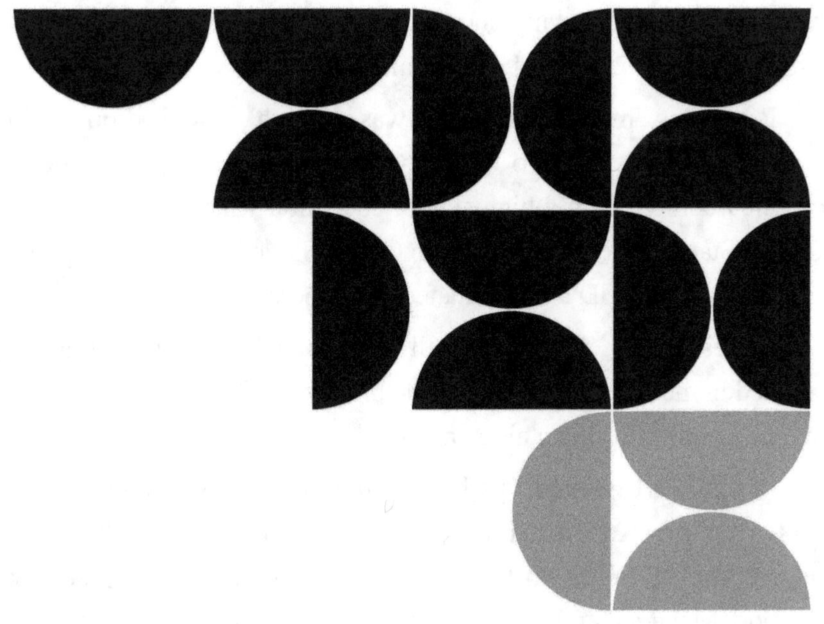

ABOUT THE AUTHOR

My name is Ali Deniz Özkan, I was born in Ankara, Türkiye, in 1975. With my family, I moved to Switzerland in 1984. In 1999, I moved to San Diego, California, where I stayed for 11 and a half years. I returned to Switzerland in 2011 and, in 2017, moved to Buenos Aires, Argentina. In August 2018, I embarked on a nomadic life in Latin America. I've been living this way ever since.

My main passion in life is playing rock music. I've been playing in bands and producing original music since I was fourteen. I have played in bands in Switzerland and the United States. Since 2011, I have solely focused on my one-person band, Black Sea Storm, which I founded in 2002 in San Diego, California.

Regarding my education, I was a high school dropout in Switzerland. I decided to quit school to focus on my rock music career. I completed my high school education when I moved to the United States. I went to San Diego City College for three years, then transferred to UCSD and graduated from there in 2008 with a BA.

Professionally, I have had all kinds of jobs. In Switzerland, I worked in meat and watch factories, briefly in a Turkish kebab shop, and as an educator in an elementary school.

In the US, I worked as a barista in coffee shops and managed a mid-sized Mexican restaurant for a few years. After getting my degree from UCSD, I worked in the software industry as a Customer Support Manager and then as a Director of Operations. I've done some freelance work as a software tester and linguist remotely while living in Latin America.

In 2024, I became a Solopreneur, created an LLC in New Mexico, USA, and obtained residency in Paraguay. I have wanted to be an entrepreneur for a long time, and finally, in 2024, the stars aligned for me.

Since I arrived in Latin America, I have had the opportunity to live in Argentina, Chile, Uruguay, Paraguay, Peru, Colombia, Guatemala, and Mexico. In Mexico alone, I lived in 23 different cities.

I speak four languages fluently, which is a big plus when traveling and researching information. Nowadays, it is tough to find the truth. Knowing many languages allows me to cross-check information and points of view on global topics to form my own opinion.

At the end of 2015, I got my second divorce and lost my job soon after. During that period, when I was looking for a new job opportunity, I discovered fasting. It was a turning point in my life. Besides making me healthier, fasting made me face the fact that I was unhappy in Switzerland and had to do something about it. It was essential in my decision to leave Switzerland for good and move to Latin America. It also guided me toward a nomadic life after living in Argentina for a year and a half.

Since I started fasting, I feel younger every year. I don't relate to my chronological age. I not only feel younger physically but also mentally. I embrace new technological trends and am not afraid to start new things. I can learn any new skill.

I go to the gym five to six times a week. I don't have any significant health issues. I enjoy life as much as I can. As I am writing this, I have been living out of my backpacks for the past eight years in hostels and Airbnbs. I've been constantly adapting to new environments for all those years, which does not tire me. On the contrary, it makes me feel stronger.

Eventually, I turned my nomadic life into a rock-n-roll tour in Latin America, playing solo shows in many countries. In 2022, I was able to tour Türkiye with my band, Black Sea Storm. Black Sea Storm played 21 concerts in the country. Touring is one of the most challenging things for the human metabolism. I am blown away by how much better I can cope with touring nowadays than 15 years ago. I am fifteen years older, but somehow, I am stronger and more resilient when confronted with challenges.

I love my current life and fight daily to make it sustainable.

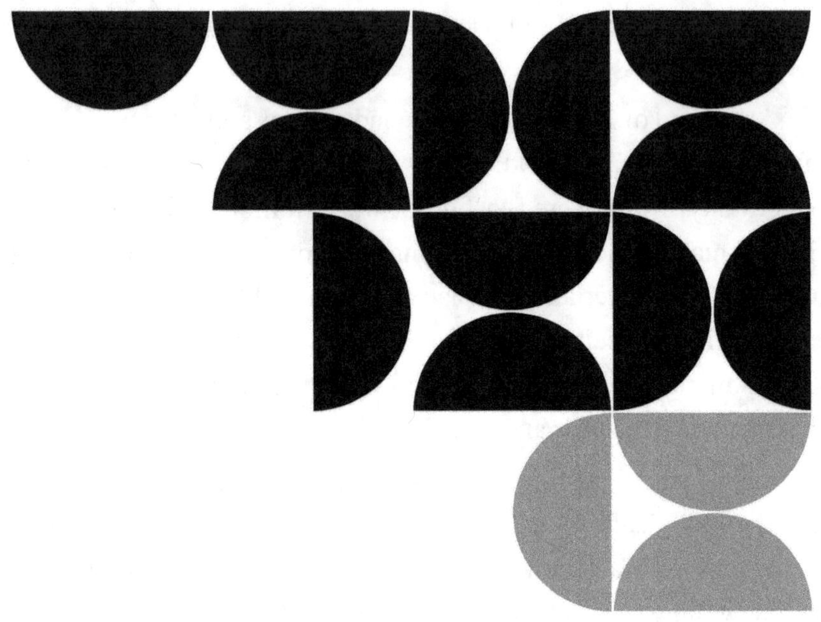

THE HEALTH ISSUES I EXPERIENCED BEFORE I STARTED FASTING

While I was a child living in Ankara, I would get sick often. The air pollution in major Turkish cities was considerable in the late '70s and early '80s, and Ankara gets very cold in the winter. My mother was into modern medicine back then. She took the doctors' authority very seriously. For about four years, I would get allergy shots at the hospital every week; if I had a cold or sore throat, my mom would give me medicine. Occasionally my grandpa, who was a paramedic in the Turkish Army, would come and provide me with penicillin shots in the butt when I was more severely sick.

When I woke up, I felt dizzy and tired, as if I had been drugged. I'd constantly be yawning during the day. Comparing my early days on Earth with how I feel now is just mind-blowing to me. I was an old, sick man back then, but now I am a healthy young kid with a ton of energy. Although socially, I had a great life when I was a child in Ankara, health-wise, it was a disaster.

When we moved with my family to Switzerland in the mid-'80s, we lived in a Swiss village, so it was a far better situation regarding air pollution. My mom's fetish for modern medicine continued there. I would get sick occasionally, but playing in nature, riding my bike, and doing various sports helped my health considerably. Socially, I struggled a lot during the first couple of years and missed Ankara. Eventually, I learned French and started to make friends in Switzerland.

Back then, I had a Coca-Cola addiction and would eat at McDonald's a lot.

The first major health issue I had in Switzerland was inflammation and pain in my right arm. Back then, I played tennis a lot. I quit tennis around 14 and started playing guitar, then bass guitar. I was obsessed with playing rock music. I was making good progress until the tendon problems I had with tennis flared up again. And now I had the issue on both arms. At one point, the doctor told me to take a break from playing guitar. My whole world collapsed. It was tough for me not to be able to do the thing I loved the most.

After trying everything possible according to modern medicine, my mom told me she had seen an osteopath and had great results. In the early '90s in Switzerland, osteopaths weren't expected to challenge modern medicine and the dominant ideology. I was very skeptical of the whole osteopath thing at first.

I had the idea that the osteopath was going to be a Chaman-type healer. I was ignorant. My mom ended up convincing me to see him. The osteopath fixed my arms enough to the point where I was back playing in bands. But I needed to be very careful not to inflame my tendons. I will wear tennis bands, and inflammation will reappear if I play for over two or three hours. It was so frustrating. I wanted to give it my all to rock n' roll, but the tendon issue kept me from playing as much as I wanted.

However, despite my slight handicap, I played in many bands, was able to go on many tours, and released albums. I would always wear tennis armbands to delay any possible inflammation.

When I started fasting regularly in 2016, the inflammation disappeared within a year. I stopped wearing the tennis armbands around 2018. Now, I can play for as many hours as I like without thinking about inflaming my tendons.

Resolving the tendon inflammation was the most prominent and immediate result of fasting, but it was far from the only issue my body could fix. I was suffering from kidney pain, psoriasis, eczema, and hemorrhoids. My digestion was so-so. At times, I would have urges to pee for no apparent reason. I would experience small muscular injuries. Fasting took away all these minor but uncomfortable symptoms from my life. When I remember these conditions, it feels like I was from a different life.

Besides the tendon problems, all my health issues were minor. But who knows, if I hadn't fixed them, they could have become more severe with time. Thanks to fasting, I gained flexibility and endurance; I can go to the gym more often. Every year since I started fasting, I feel younger, and I have more overall enthusiasm. I am so disconnected from my chronological age.

For all those reasons, I am responsible for sharing my experience with others. Health issues should not keep us from achieving our true potential and focusing on our purpose in life.

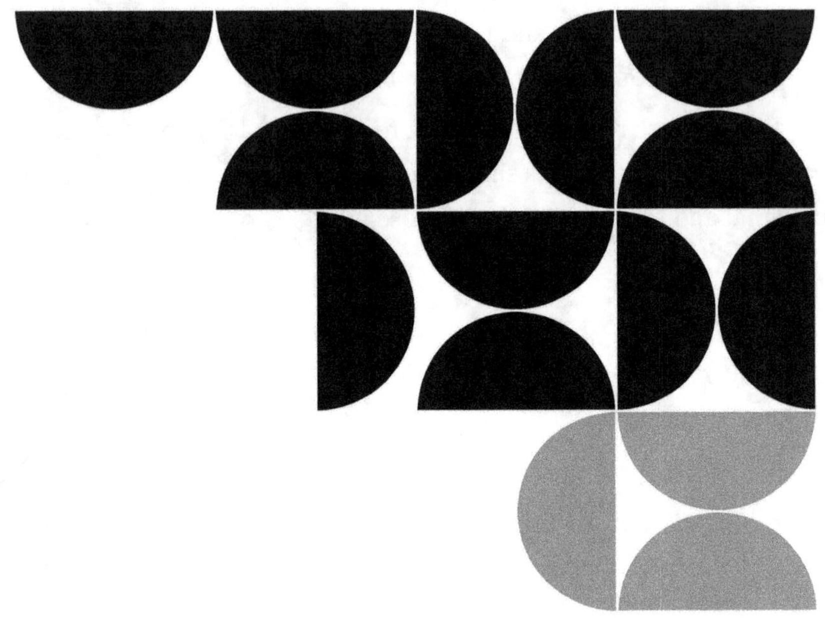

THE THINGS FASTING MADE ME QUIT

With fasting entering my life in 2016, I started to quit certain addictions and bad habits. The first addiction I got rid of was alcohol. I did quit drinking pretty much at the same time as I began fasting. About a year after starting the fasting journey, I quit all medicinal drugs. Later on, in 2018, I stopped drinking coffee until 2024. I had a lousy coffee addiction. I would drink between eight to ten cups a day. Taking a long break from coffee was very beneficial to me. I've recently made my return to drink coffee. I can enjoy the beverage with more moderation now.

Since 2017, I haven't had medical insurance. It's, of course, a risk, and I don't recommend it. In case of an accident, it could be a problem, but with any other medical condition that is not mechanical, I have faith that I can fix it with fasting. When I lived in Switzerland, I had the cheapest insurance policy possible, which still cost me 4000 Swiss Francs a year. It has now been over eight years since I have lived without insurance. The money I have saved is at least over 32,000 Swiss francs. Since insurance costs also rise as we age, I have saved even more money.

Even if I had a significant accident in Latin America, I'd probably pull it off with a lesser amount in medical bills. It's a bet I took. I don't recommend it, but I am thrilled with my decision. Not only have I saved a ton of cash, but most importantly, I am not fueling an industry I don't believe in.

I quit using conventional toothpaste. I am geared toward natural alternatives; occasionally, I make my own with coconut oil mixed with baking soda.

I quit using cosmetics such as day cream, night cream, body lotions, etc., and I stopped using fragrances for about seven years. I started using some again in 2023, but I avoid using fragrance too often on my skin. I'll instead put it on my T-shirt.

I quit using some natural hair lotions that would slow down my hair loss. The lotions worked well, but I stopped using them for financial reasons. I knew I would be living in Latin America soon, and it would be difficult for me to keep buying such products made in Switzerland.

Before I started fasting, I was already capable of quitting bad habits. I was able to quit smoking and quit putting sugar in my coffee. In 2002, I stopped watching regular TV. It was at first a political stand. I used to live in the US back then. After September 2001, American TV turned into an anti-Muslim propaganda machine. I decided not to give my money to those people. Still, to this day, it is one of the best decisions I have made in life.

Between 2017 and 2021, I managed to live without a cell phone plan. I am still trying to figure out how I pulled that one off, but I did. When I arrived in Guatemala in 2021, I bought a SIM card. I lived in Argentina, Uruguay, Mexico, Chile, and Peru without a cellphone plan. For some reason, I perceived Guatemala as more dangerous than other places I had traveled to without a cell phone plan, so I decided to break the SIM fast. To this day, I buy local SIMs wherever I go.

More recently, in 2023, I started a ketogenic diet. I no longer consume processed sugars and quit eating bread, pasta, potatoes, beans, lentils, etc. I also avoid fruits with high sugar and starch content, such as mangoes, bananas, grapes, and apples.

Recently, I quit using toilet paper. I've read that the chemicals used to bleach toilet paper aren't very good for our microbiota. With the keto diet, my stools have become soft and compact, which makes it very easy to clean myself. After finishing my business, I wash myself with water and soap and have a dedicated towel to dry myself. That towel I don't use is to dry my face or hands. After finishing, I wash my hands thoroughly and dry them with a different towel. And voilà.

I have also quit using seed oils. When we eat out, knowing what kind of oil the restaurant uses becomes more challenging. Since I have cooked almost all my meals since I started keto, I have better control over the oil situation.

The next thing I want to quit is using harmful cookware such as Teflon pans, black plastic spatulas, and plastic cutting boards. Being a nomad makes it challenging to travel with pans and casseroles, but as I write this, I am in the process of getting a residency in Paraguay. Even if I don't stay here all year round, I plan on getting storage and putting my heavy things there. This new situation will allow me to buy the appropriate cookware. In Airbnb, the kitchen items are often of poor quality in Latin America. I travel with my kitchen knives, cutting board, strainer, and gloves for dishes, but I still have to rely on what is available for heavy items.

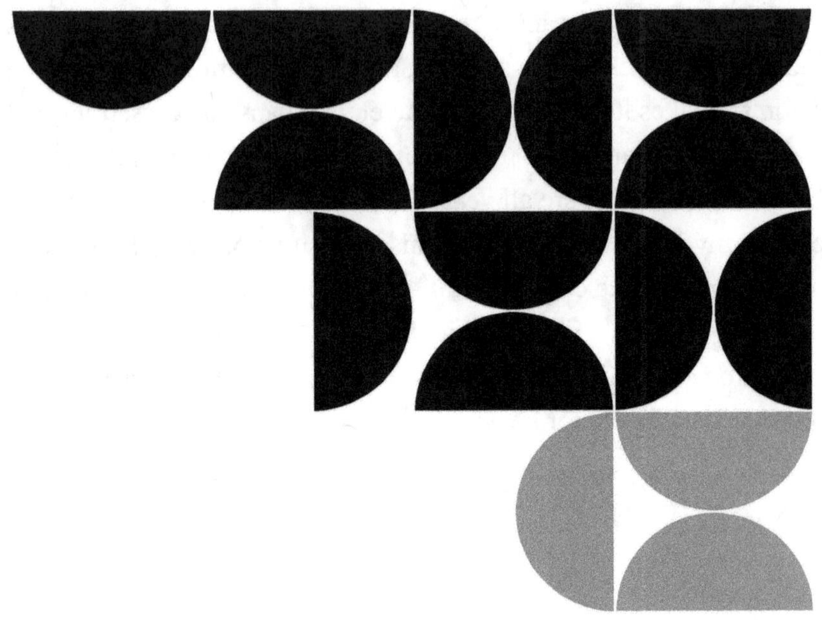

HOW FASTING CHANGED MY LIFE

If I had to divide my time on this planet into two, there was my life before I started fasting and my life after.

Fasting changed my life for the better. The first nine months of fasting had a powerful effect on improving my physical health. My digestion improved, and I was able to get rid of tendon inflammation, skin problems, kidney pain, allergies, and hemorrhoids. I started sleeping better. I hadn't gotten injured with minor muscular injuries as before.

After nine months, I started to feel that fasting was affecting me mentally. I had some mental healing crises during extended fasts, and I would weep out crying intensely. I was able to recover from past traumas this way. I also did a mental cleanse where almost all my goals in life collapsed. Only my love for music and the soccer team I root for have survived. This mental flush was the scariest part of fasting for me. For a while, I felt goalless in life. But with time, I had new goals more aligned with my true self.

I then started questioning my life's purpose and mission on this planet. Answering those questions allowed me to align everything I do with my purpose. I also got closer to my faith. I found that what I discovered with fasting was already in my religion. So, I looked at my faith in a different light and decided to practice it more.

Fasting allowed me to have better physical health, make better decisions, stop lying to myself, and be aligned with my purpose.

It is still an ongoing process. Finding who we are may be our mission on this planet.

Since 2016, fasting has become a lifestyle for me. It is a practice that guides me through life.

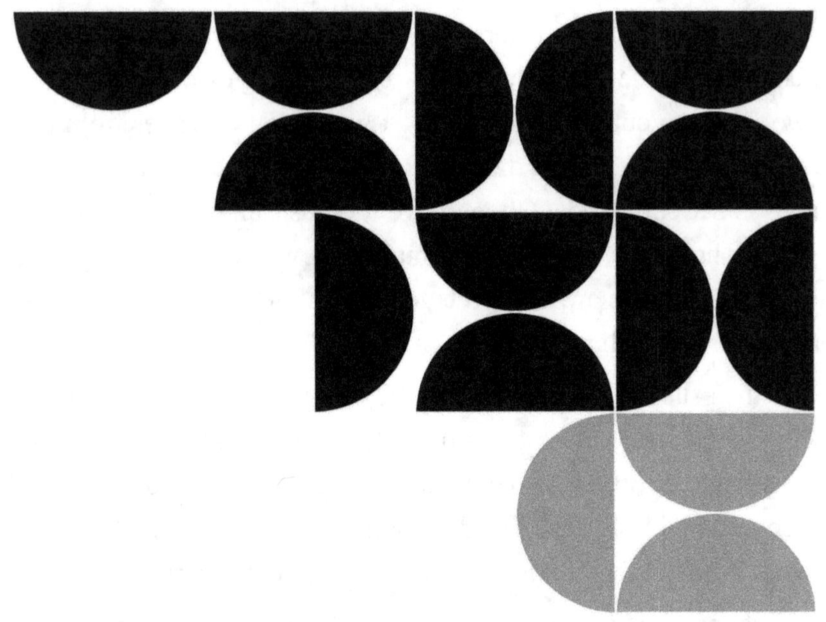

I LIVE MY FASTING EXPERIENCE AS A JOURNEY

Fasting is not a diet. Although it requires a certain amount of discipline, it's not a continuous set routine. Fasting triggers cleansing, reconstruction, and rejuvenation mechanisms within our body, consequently bringing change. We need to keep an open mind to this change and adapt to keep progressing.

It's like the surfer riding a wave. To reach stability and ride the wave, the surfer must constantly adapt to changing factors; if she does not, a fall will occur. This is why, with fasting, we need to learn to listen to what our bodies are trying to express through symptoms and feelings.

Fasting should always be exciting. If not, we must rest from fasting or challenge our bodies even more. We want to get to a point where we are excited to go into a fast, and we are excited to go back to our comfort zone. That way, we keep the excitement alive. It's like traveling. It excited us to go on vacation, and returning home felt good. We will move forward in our journey by going back and forth with moments of stress and relaxation.

Yes, fasting is a journey because if we fast regularly, our experiences evolve. What we felt on the third day of a fast may not occur on the third day of the next fast. There is a sense of making progress with fasting regularly, so it feels like a big journey. This journey, like any adventure, makes fasting incredibly exciting.

Fasting tends to improve every function within our body and mind. This improvement creates a sense of self-actualization for me. I want to go back to fasting to discover new frontiers when I go back to my comfort zone after a fast and notice the positive change; I want to go back to fasting soon so I can keep moving forward and become a better version of myself, thanks to my fasting journey.

As I write this, it has been eight years since I incorporated fasting into my life. I still have only completed five percent of the fasting journey. This feeling comes from a sense that there's still room for improvement and eventually becoming the better version of myself.

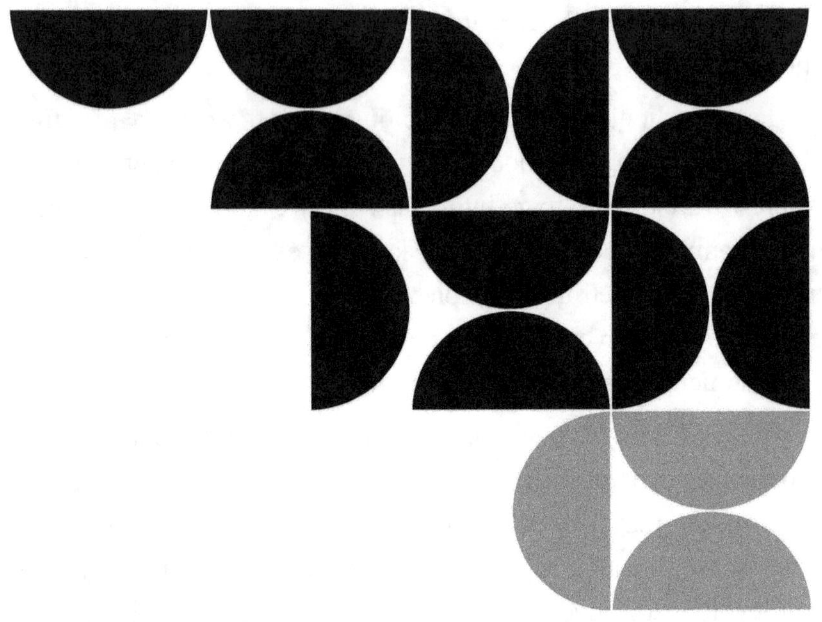

FASTING FOR A BETTER MONDAY

Where does the title of this book come from? *For a Better Monday* is based on the title of a song I wrote with my ex-band, Channing Cope, in 2004. It is the closing song of our album *Sugar in Our Blood*, released the same year.

When I started my fasting experience, I felt an immense need to share it. I started a blog called *For a Better Monday*. My initial idea was to communicate that we are not fasting just for health; we want to be healthy to tackle our life's missions. I tried to convey the idea of looking forward to work on Monday.

As my life has evolved from employee to freelancer to entrepreneur, the meaning has slightly changed. If you don't like your Mondays, change your life until you look forward to them. I am personally going after this pursuit. Since 2017, I have lived in Latin America; since 2018, I have lived a nomadic life and love all days of the week. I usually work seven days a week. Mondays still have a Monday flavor because I collaborate with manufacturers and freelancers, and they are mainly on a weekly schedule. I love everything I do, so work no longer feels like work.

It fascinates me that with Channing Cope, we released a song called "For A Better Monday," and the album title is *Sugar in Our Blood*. Back then, I had no interest in fasting or human physiology. The fact that "For A Better Monday" is in the *Sugar in Our Blood* album is one of those signs that life throws at us, and we only understand later on. Back then, it did not occur that if we controlled the sugar in our blood, we would access a better Monday. It's an interesting coincidence; somehow, the unconscious mind can express itself through music and art.

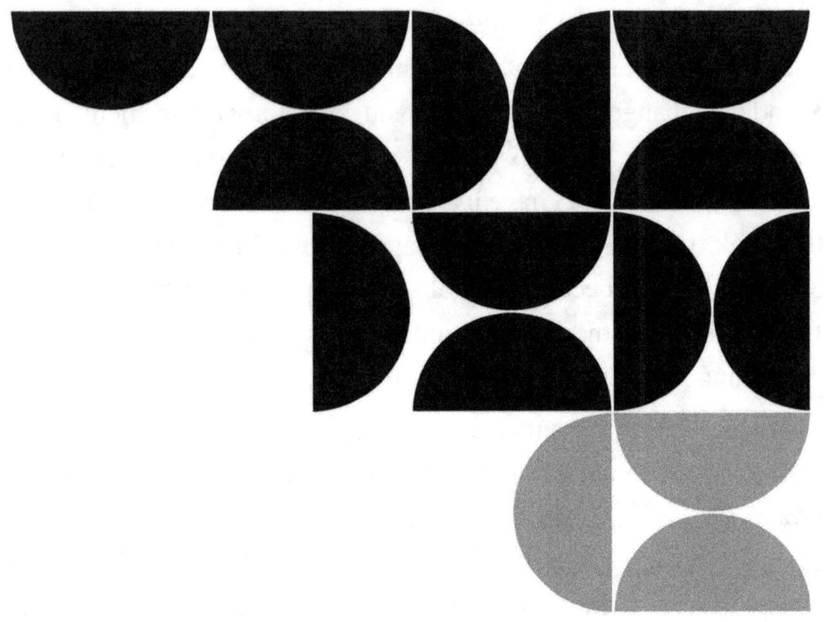

THE STORY OF MY HAIR AND FASTING MY SCALP

In this chapter, I want to discuss the history of my hair and how fasting helped me solve scalp-related issues. The information in this chapter is very personal, but the history of my hair and scalp gives good insight into the evolution of my overall health. That is why I wanted to share this information with you.

I had soft, straight, shiny, good-quality black hair as a child. When I hit puberty and went through hormonal changes, I started to have some scalp problems. My scalp would either be too dry or too greasy. I had way too much hair. During my metal head years, I would shave the sides and back of my head in Jason Newsted's style. If I didn't, the volume of my long black hair would be out of control.

I tried all kinds of shampoo and could not solve my scalp problem. Around my twenties, I started to lose my hair. I saw an ad in the local newspaper for a local Swiss clinic that specialized in hair treatment. The ad looked like a scam, but I decided to try it.

I went to the clinic several times a week for six months. They applied some natural hair lotion to my scalp, and beautiful Brazilian ladies massaged it so the solution would penetrate the scalp. The hair loss slowed considerably, and the quality of my hair improved. The most important part was that my scalp felt and smelled amazing. Contrary to appearances, the whole thing was not a scam. It worked!

Once the six-month treatment was over, they told me that if I wanted to maintain my current status, I had to apply some of the lotions myself at home. It was a considerable investment of time and money, but the results were there, so I consistently applied the products in the morning and at night. Believe it or not, from the mid-'90s to 2016, I used those natural hair products. When I moved to the US, my mom continued to send them to me from Switzerland every six months for over a decade! Turkish moms are great like that!

In 2016, when I got into fasting and prepared for my departure for Latin America, I knew that with my new life standards, I could not afford the relatively expensive artisanal Swiss lotions. So, I decided to quit the lotions. My scalp quickly returned to having the too dry, too greasy situation. I tried all kinds of shampoos, and I would get some results for a short period, and then I would be back to experiencing an imbalance in my scalp.

Since I started my fasting journey, I have applied a similar approach to shampooing my hair. I washed my hair with shampoo three to four times a week but decided to space the time between shampoo use. I started washing my hair with shampoo twice a week, then once. I then started washing my hair every ten days, fifteen days, twenty days, and thirty days.

At one point, I stopped using shampoo altogether.

From my understanding, the human scalp is a surface where bacteria, yeast, and fungi live together in an equilibrium, feeding off each other. If we exterminate one group, for instance, with antifungal shampoo, we break the equilibrium between the three groups, and we may experience uncontrolled growth in the remaining two groups. In my case, using Swiss lotion first and then fasting my scalp helped the situation. My overall fasting journey also affected the situation positively.

I have dyed my hair since I moved to the US in 1999. Back then, I had one or two gray hairs. On my first visit, my first hairdresser in Pacific Beach in San Diego, California, asked me, "Do you want me to cover your grays?" I said okay. Since then, I have become accustomed to covering my grays whenever I go to the hairdresser.

I believed I only had a few gray hairs as the years passed. After losing my job and starting to make plans to move to Argentina in 2016, I decided to cut down on all the unnecessary expenses. So, I purchased a hair clipper and shaved my head. Surprisingly, I noticed I had way more gray hair than I thought. I was in shock. Since getting into fasting, I have researched demineralization, and I learned one of the earliest signs of demineralization is starting to have gray hair. Seeing that my gray hair situation got to an advanced stage without me noticing made me feel like I had missed the natural warning signs my body was sending me.

While living in Switzerland, I shaved my hair and did not dye it. As I approached my departure, I started growing and dyeing my hair again. I wanted to psychologically feel the best I could before beginning this new chapter of my life in South America. Once I arrived in Buenos Aires, I stopped dying my hair. The idea was not to use toxic products to support my fasting journey positively.

Up until November 2018, I did not dye my hair. While in Oaxaca, México, I met a beautiful woman online. When the opportunity came to visit her in Querétaro for a first date, I decided to dye my hair before the trip to put all the chances of seducing her on my side. It worked; I went out with her for almost two years. Since then, I have been dying my hair. From a purely health angle, not dyeing my hair would be better. Since I stopped using cosmetics altogether, it would make more sense not to dye my hair. Visually, I like myself better with my original hair color. As I get older, I may stop dyeing my hair, but for now, I am comfortable with the compromise.

I still very rarely shampoo my hair. If I go to the hairdresser to dye my hair, they wash it with shampoo. If I dye my hair at home, I don't use shampoo or natural solid shampoo.

The scalp fasting worked well in fighting my too-dry/too-greasy scalp situation. Another problem I had for many years, and I do not remember when it started, was that my scalp produced flake-like skin particles. It drove me crazy because it would sometimes go away or intensify depending on where I was during my travels and what I ate. It might have something to do with the fungi bacteria yeast balance, but I could not understand what affected the situation.

Once I started the ketogenic diet, I was able to determine the root cause. Since then, the flake-like skin production problem has almost disappeared 100%! I am unsure if my body was getting rid of the excess sugar through my scalp; one thing I am sure of is a correlation between sugar, carbs, and the production of these skin particles.

Unfortunately, my hair loss has increased since I stopped using the lotions in 2016. Although keto is also positively affecting my hair loss situation, I've been getting to a point where it is more visible that I am losing my hair. Since I had a lot of hair, even though I've been losing my hair since my twenties, nobody noticed.

The last time I was in Türkiye, my parents separately offered me a hair transplant operation as a gift. It made me smile that they had the same idea without consulting each other. The hair transplant business is pretty unique in Türkiye. I've seen mind-blowing results.

I am considering it next time I return to Türkiye, but I have some concerns about using antibiotics. Since I quit medication, antibiotics are the last thing I want to put in my body. Also, I want to know if I can still dye my transplanted hair. One other factor that is turning me off is that we need to stop sports and exercising for a month after the operation. With my current lifestyle, stopping exercising for a month is unthinkable. And if, on top of that, I need to take antibiotics, it's a terrible combination without saying that in Türkiye, secondhand smoke is widespread and intense. So, the whole Turkish hair transplant cocktail would be taking me away from the healthy lifestyle I am trying to build myself day after day.

The easiest solution might be to accept to be a bald but healthy guy.

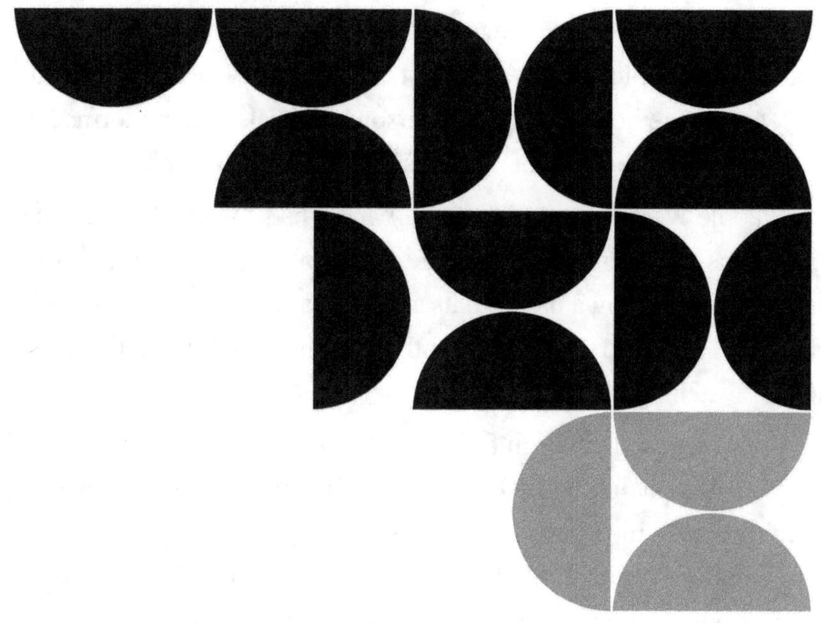

WHAT CONVINCED ME TO ACCEPT TO BUILD BUSINESSES AROUND MY FASTING EXPERIENCE

A year after I started fasting, I had the burning desire to share my experience. I could not believe the transformation I was experiencing. I was suffering less at all levels. I started a blog for-a-better-monday.com to share my experience with others. Whenever I met someone, I couldn't stop talking about fasting.

In 2018, I embraced the nomadic life, which allowed me to meet many new people wherever I went. In addition, I was putting little rock tours together with my one-person band, Black Sea Storm. That activity also gave me a lot of exposure to meet new people.

People were very interested in what I had to say about fasting, but it was sometimes challenging to convince them. Although I did not consider fasting a passion, its ability to allow me to self-actualize made me obsessed. I was constantly thinking about it, reading about it, and watching YouTube videos.

I asked myself if I could earn money as a fasting coach. I would be more convincing if I had nothing to sell. I went from town to town, playing music, meeting people, and spreading the word about fasting. At one point, I even thought that God gave me rock n' roll not to sell records but as a carrot to make me move around the globe and spread the good word. I had a very romantic approach to what I was doing.

The incredible thing was that when people messaged me with questions about fasting, I would stop what I was doing and thoroughly answer them with DMs or voicemails. It did not feel like work, and I didn't feel like I was missing out on other things. My duty as a human being was to pass on this message so people would stop suffering and focus on their life's purpose.

For years, making money with fasting was out of the question. Late in 2023, I got sick of doing freelance work and asking my family for financial support when I couldn't make ends meet. I decided to become a seller on Amazon to reach financial independence. I signed up for an online course from a very successful French entrepreneur. I barely completed 25% of the course when a mentorship opportunity opened within the same community. I accepted the free call with a mentor named Livio. Right on the free call, Livio saved me a lot of time and trouble with my plan to start a business.

We started the mentoring program. Our goal was to find a niche product to sell on Amazon. Livio took the time to get to know me, my passions, and my hobbies. He let me research my niche on Amazon for a couple of weeks. I spent a lot of time on the site with the Helium 10 plugin. I came up with several ideas. I would present them to Livio, and he would find the weak points in my findings and tell me that they did not qualify for a proper niche product.

I was learning a lot but needed to be more successful at finding a product. One day, I presented my new findings, and Livio trashed them all and then said, "Okay. Enough playing. I have a good niche product for you that aligns with your passion for fasting." The actual product was perfect. There were only two main competitors, and they were generating a lot of money with their products. However, there was still a lot of room for improvement.

I was impressed that the solution was right in front of my nose, but I did not see the opportunity since I wanted to make money with something other than fasting. I briefly shared my thoughts about not being willing to make money from fasting with Livio. However, he convinced me otherwise. He told me that I had great faith in fasting being an activity that could better society and that I should use the power of capitalism to amplify the message and reach way more people than I would touring with my band and talking to few people here and there about fasting.

It was a genius touch from Livio. Not only did he provide me with a fantastic niche product, but most importantly, he aligned me even more with my true purpose in life. Even if the product did not work, I knew I wanted to be in the fasting business. That way, I could solve all my problems and others' problems.

The big lesson I learned about the whole experience was that investing in knowledge is very important. Investing money into the course and mentoring saved me a great deal of time and provided the final touch in my life alignment. It motivated me to be successful in business and be able to invest more in mentoring in the future.

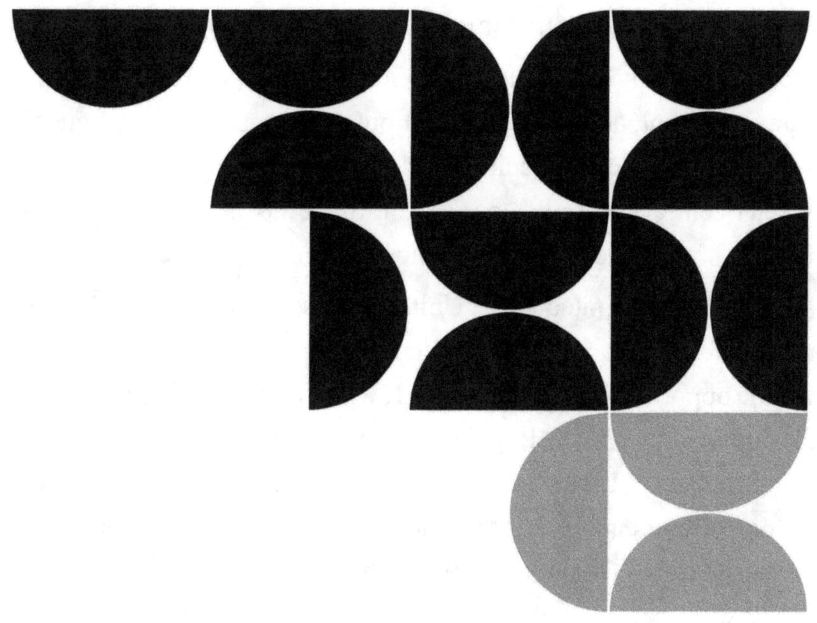

HOW FASTING GOT ME CLOSER TO MY FAITH

I was born in a very secular Turkish family. My parents did not practice Islam as far as I know but considered themselves Muslim. My entire family on both sides is Muslim, but during the '70s, '80s, and '90s, secularism was very dominant in Türkiye, especially in the environment where I grew up. I did not think much about religion growing up. When we made it to Switzerland, I had a childhood friend with no religion, and I thought it would be cool to be like him. In my teenage years, I realized that having no religion wasn't for me, so I identified myself as being Muslim. Besides praying and unconventionally connecting with God, I did not practice Islam at all. I drank alcohol, ate pork, and went out with many women. I guess I was what they call a cultural Muslim. Religion and spirituality weren't central to my life back then. Since nobody seemed to care much at home about religion, nothing pushed me to practice my faith.

In 1999, I migrated to the United States from Switzerland. It was an excellent move for me. I wanted to live the American dream and had the opportunity to do so. In 2001, while I was living in San Diego, California, September 11th happened. I thought, "What a terrible terrorist attack." I was convinced that the US agencies would catch the perpetrators and bring them to justice. My reference for feeling that way was the Oklahoma City bombing. Things did not evolve that way at all. Very soon, the US president declared the country at war. The US invaded Afghanistan and then Iraq. I was thinking that after the attacks of September 11th, the media would talk about the terrible event for a few weeks, and then it would be business as usual. That did not happen as I thought it would, either. The theme of Islamist terrorism and being at war never went away.

Slowly, the anti-terrorist sentiment was becoming an anti-Muslim sentiment. As if the two were interchangeable. The US mainstream media became an anti-Muslim propaganda machine.

I could not watch TV anymore. After the 2002 Soccer World Cup, I decided to cancel my cable membership. I started to say aloud that I was a Muslim, even though I wasn't practicing.

I played in rock bands, attended San Diego City College, and worked at local coffee shops. I wanted to show people that Muslims are very diverse and that you can be a rocker, a barista, a college student, and a Muslim at the same time.

During this entire time, the anti-Muslim propaganda was spreading in the United States. Not once did I experience racism. I went on tours in the Midwest; I had a solid social life in San Diego. I was telling everyone I was a Muslim, and not once did somebody say or do something terrible to me. I think this is the beauty and strength of American society. It welcomes anyone. If you live in the United States, in people's heads, you are an American. At least it was that way for me while I lived in the United States.

Between 2001 and 2016, I lived as a cultural Muslim. In 2016, I started my fasting journey. I began to quit alcohol and started exercising more. I soon realized that the practices I had to embrace to reach better health were already part of my espoused faith. So, I decided to take a closer look at Islam. In 2017, I fasted my first Ramadan and started to read the Holy Quran. I would do Ramadan every year and get closer to my religion during that month. In 2023, near the end of Ramadan, I started praying five times a day. I cannot always keep it up or do it on time, but in the weeks and months when I pray five times a day, everything works better for me.

To sum up, my relationship with fasting and my faith is that most Muslims fast because of their religion. Even though I was born Muslim, fasting got me closer to Islam, not the other way around. My fasting experience proved that my religion was the right path to becoming a better human being.

I am far from following all the rules of Islam, but fasting and praying have already been highly beneficial to me. I intend to become a better Muslim step by step without forcing myself, but I will embrace each practice when I feel ready. Islam has captured something true about the human body, mind, and spirituality. Only good things will happen to me if I follow this path. It feels like when I make one step toward God, He makes ten toward me.

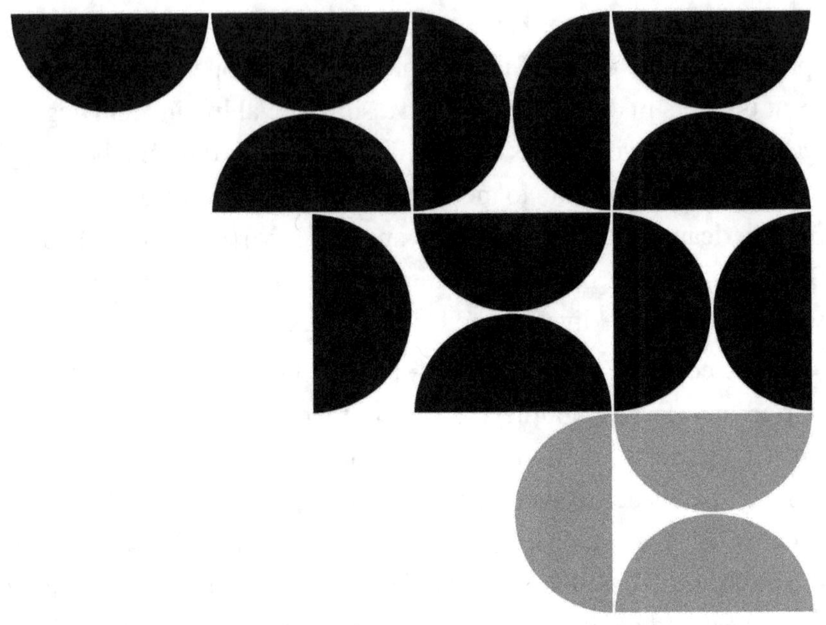

THE NEXT STEPS I WANT TO TAKE

While predicting the future is impossible, I'm excited about the possibilities. After releasing this book, I'm eager to take the next steps forward on my fasting journey and contribute to a healthier future.

My journey with fasting began in 2016, and it was a transformative experience. Fasting solved most of my problems, and I want to share this journey with others. I aim to develop an understanding of how fasting can work for individuals with different profiles, just as it did for me.

With my brand, Better Monday Fasting, I am planning on starting coaching. With the information I will gather from this coaching experience, I plan to become a better coach and incorporate my learnings into future books on fasting or new editions of *For A Better Monday*.

The first chapter of this book is called "There Is No Set Formula or Protocol for Fasting." I still believe in this idea, but if I gain experience working with people with different physiological profiles, we could develop an approach where, depending on the profile type, there is a custom-made protocol for that person.

As I wrote the last chapter of this book, I connected with a person looking for a fasting coach. I am excited to accompany this person on his fasting journey and to learn more about fasting through someone else's experience.

I also have some ideas for digital products related to fasting. I want to develop them and launch them under my brand, Better Monday Fasting.

With my other brand, YouthLyte, I plan to launch my first physical product, Fasting Electrolytes, in November 2024. The product will only be available on Amazon US to get us started. I have other physical product ideas that support fasting in the pipeline; depending on the first product's success, I will launch more items on the YouthLyte Amazon store.

Everything should come together nicely in 2025. This book and the related digital and physical products will hopefully create an excellent arsenal to accompany us on our fasting journey.

I have also started an X account for Better Monday Fasting (@BetterMFasting). I want to build an audience interested in fasting.

We can share our knowledge and experience on that medium and learn more about fasting. I plan on growing on X before eventually tackling other social media platforms. I enjoy the silent and minimal aspect of X.

Through the various projects I launch, I am committed to continuously learning about fasting. I aim to integrate my new learnings into my fasting journey, getting closer to becoming the best version of myself and reaching 100% health. I want to create a virtuous circle where I learn, experiment, get feedback, and positively impact society. Although my fasting journey started in 2016, it feels like the most exciting part of the adventure is about to begin.